Introduction

Reading the books on autoimmune and ways of reversing it have really intrigued me. I wanted to educate myself on what would be best for me and my family. Having an autistic son and a son who has acne, allergies, and asthma, I needed to see if I could help combat some of the issues and prevent anything else from occurring.

I adopted the vegan-seafood-gluten free diet starting September 1, 2017. Of course, this was a lot harder to follow than I predicted, and I wasn't getting the results I wanted. I knew I needed a better solution.

During the Super bowl (2018), my youngest son went to our friend's party and ate everything he wasn't supposed too. He came home super hyper, unfocused, and not listening. We couldn't even get him to stop and listen to the directions we were giving him. I was not able to attend the party, due to having a "flare" day (thanks to Addison's Disease and Fibromyalgia), had I been there, he would not have had the "no-no" foods.

I read *Food Over Medicine* and then dived into the *Autoimmune Solution*. Giving me the idea to track this new diet, get it down, and see what my progress is and if I can help others. I wanted to know if this really works, and if the disease can be reversed. Since these books take on a few different points of views from different doctors, it was hard to try and follow each one like the books stated. I liked what they were saying but needed to take in what my body was already doing from the diet I've been on. I knew I wanted to stick with a whole food plant-based diet, moving away from seafood, but I also knew the benefits of bone broth, so I wanted to incorporate that as well. Getting through a few more books as I went along with this new plan, I was able to tweak what needed to be tweaked, but stayed on the whole food plant-based plan. I tracked my symptoms as well as my youngest son's behavior and focus, and my older son's Acne and allergies. Since my oldest son isn't with me full time, I can't really track his progress. Instead, for him, we took him off of dairy for 30 days. It was one simple thing and easy for him to do when he was with his dad.

Starting a 50-day plan and sticking to it is was my goal. I tracked it day by day, symptoms, energy, intake of food and

beverage, exercise, medicines, activity level, and Dr. appointments. All of it. The good the bad and the ugly.

I wanted this to come from someone who had no medical background, just someone with 2 autoimmune diseases and low back issues. At the end of 50 days, I could better determine how this WFPB diet could really help and if it was able to reverse the diseases that I have.

30 days didn't feel like enough time for me to get enough information from the WFPB diet.

I started with what I had around the house, if it was canned (like beans) I used it up and then went and bought a bag of beans. I had over processed pasta and bread, which are gluten free, but looked for more organic less processed brands and didn't worry if it was gluten free or not. With moving away from the gluten free, I was worried that we might have a "reaction" of some sort. If our bodies didn't handle the non-gluten free things, we would move back to doing gluten free. Instead of buying bread, I started making my own. I planned on meal prepping 2-3 times a week, if I had the energy, and go from there.

This WFPB plan is based on the 2 autoimmune diseases that I have, Addison's and Fibro, and for chronic low back pain/inflammation. I can't speak for any other autoimmune diseases because I don't have them, so this is would be considered my "specialty" and what worked for my diseases, health level, and body type.

One of the books I read talked about limiting oils, especially if you are in it for weight loss, which I was not. I did use a lot less oils but did not eliminate them completely. Another book I read, praises bone broth and how healing it can be to leaky gut, but I wanted to keep this WFPB, so I decided that I would just leave it out for now and just keep it vegan for the 50 days.

This is my journey through 50 days of the WFPB diet. I hope you learn from my experience and it inspires you one way or another.

First day Thoughts

People want to feel better and say they will change so they can start seeing results. Unless it involves food.

"Oh, I don't want to take more pills. I don't' like the side effect and how they make me feel."

Ok! So, change the way you eat.

"But I like food."

No one said become anorexic and never eat again. Just change your diet and take out the foods that are making you sick.

"But I can't live without dairy, breads, sugars…. But, but, but"

Ok, so what I'm hearing is that you would rather be in pain and feel shitty and slowly die because the foods that are making you feel this way, you can't live without…Hmmm. Does this make sense? If the food on this plan will help give you a better life, would you do it?

Trust me (someone who thought they couldn't live without a certain food), you can live a lot better without it. I haven't had milk in about 7 years. I was a milk addict. Like really. I was obsessed with milk. I, by myself went through about a gallon a day. When I had to take it out of my diet, I thought I would die. That was the end of my perfect life. No more dunking Oreos, no more ice-cold milk after a long run, no more cake and milk. All the recipes were going to suck because I couldn't' use my precious milk. My world as I had known, had ended.

Here I am; still alive. What I did notice was that my skin cleared up significantly. I didn't have the stomach bloat I had always had and could never get rid of. I felt a lot better. I bitched and moaned for about a year about it, but I couldn't deny the results. Now, I can't even look at milk. It's like looking a jug full of lard. It really turns me off. I'm not a huge fan of almond milk, but I do love me some rice milk. That shit is good.

I will be tracking what my 9-year-old son is eating as well. He is going to do the WFPB plan with me. I want to see if it helps him focus a bit more. He is high functioning autistic and has ADHD. We have never medicated him but when we took him off gluten and dairy…HOLY MOTHER OF GOD!! It made a HUGE difference in his behavior. Now we have been way more laxed with him because he goes to friends houses and we don't expect them to stick with the "diet." But now I will be sending him with food, because that kid is uncontrollable when he has gluten and dairy. It's like giving him crack.

I also asked my 18-year-old son to stop eating dairy for 30 days. He has allergies (to the point I want to punch him sometimes just listening to him mouth breath, because his nose is plugged 24/7), asthma, and pretty bad acne. I want to see what difference taking him off dairy will do. I am not telling him what to expect, I just asked him to do this for me for "research." He agreed, so we shall see. If he sees a difference, then I will ask him to stay off dairy for good. I am really excited to see if his acne clears up because he as Senior pictures coming up in April. Fingers crossed.

My middle son…Ok this kid must be the hulk. He never gets sick (once he had a strep infection that went undetected and he ended up in kidney failure and at the hospital for over a week, but he is good now and that has been his only sickness in his 15 years). It's like his immune system is superman and anything that enters his body his immune system says, "come at me bro" and then kicks its ass. It's truly amazing. He has really good skin for a 15-year-old boy. He has some black heads and that is it. His skin is amazing. He eats pretty shitty too. This kid should be sick a whole lot more and have the worst case of acne and allergies, but nope. He is superhuman. If I could make him change to a plant-based diet (Divorced parent, so I can't control what he eats at his dads), I would and just see how he would feel on it, athletic wise.

All 3 of my boys are super athletic so it would be pretty cool to see what they could do if they adopted a WFPB diet.

So, I have 3 different little experiments going on with 3 different types of issues. Getting this all down and the first initial steps that I will need to take to make this shit happen.

Step 1. Get all the crap out of my system

First, I need to get rid of some of the supplements I've been taking. Learning a bit more about them, I can see why there are not so great as some people might think. I mean they are made of urine and I would rather have that going out of my body than in. Birth control is another thing I need to get out of my system and I am going to miss that. I don't enjoy having periods, I am sure every woman can agree with that, so I will miss the joy of not having one. Instead I am back to facing that bitch who loves to torture my body every month with her little puranas gnawing at my stomach.

I do need to look at probiotics that are offered at my Drs. Office, they will have the best selection that health stores wouldn't get.

Step 2: Fully committing

This means getting all the shit that doesn't follow the plan out of my house, so it is not a temptation.

Step 3: The family

I do not plan on making 3 of 4 different meals to please everyone. I'm too tired and I have zero energy 98% of the time, so everyone is going to be doing the WFPB diet with me, while they are at my house. When we go to a friend's house, I will be bringing our own meals, so the temptation won't be there. My friends have always been amazing at making sure that they have food that we can have. So, this will encourage them to make a few changes themselves.

Step 4: Documenting

Documenting everything I eat (I won't be giving measurements and all that-just what I am eating and what is mainly in it) and do, how I feel, and my activity levels.

Day 1: February 6, 2018

Food consumed

Breakfast: 2 pieces of toast with peanut butter

Lunch: Salad: Cucumber, tomato, avocado, red onion, garlic, lemon juice, salt and pepper

Snack: Apple with almond butter

Dinner: Air fried tofu and red potato casserole (red potatoes, yellow onion, garlic, brussel sprouts, spinach, olive oil (tsp), turmeric, garlic salt, salt and pepper.)

Snack: None

Beverages: Water= 80 fl. oz. Spark= 10 fl. oz.

Activity level

Felt pretty good during my workout and had the energy to get it done (30 min on the elliptical and 20 min of PT routine). Though I do not suggest watching *This is us* while working out. To many feels and it really kills the energy level you need. Had to switch shows 15 min in because I wasn't wanting to cry my way through a workout.

I was active for 100 min and got in 7,124 steps.

<u>*Medicine and Vitamins*</u>

I tweaked my meds a bit since I have not felt like I am able to make it through a day. I was taking Hydrocortisone (2 pills in the am, 1 pill at noon, and 1 around 4pm.) When I was stress dosing from a recent adrenal crisis, I noticed (even though I was in crisis) I had something to get me up enough to make it to the bathroom. So, I moved my meds up a bit (3 days ago). The past 2 days I have made it through my day without struggling, needing a nap, or to rest. I am going to stay on this dose since it seems to be working for me. (3 pills in the am, 2 at noon and 1 at 4pm). I will not be adjusting my Fludrocortisone dose because my Blood pressure is doing great at the moment, so not gonna mess with a good thing.

The only vitamin I am taking at the moment is B12. I might look into a probiotic, but I am not in any hurry to do that.

<u>*Appointments*</u>

I went to therapy (or some call it counseling)… I like to call it my "bitch it out" session. Great stress reliver too (which is important in having a healthy body). It was nice to be encouraged to write this book and continue to put myself first without feeling guilty. If I don't take care of me, I won't be around to take care of them. So, never feel like you are being selfish if you want to do nice things for yourself. Do it. You deserve it. The shit our bodies put us through on a daily basis, we deserve whatever we want to help us feel better.

Energy and Symptoms

I am starting today, technically as day 1, but you have to remember that I have been veganish-seafood diet since September 1, 2017. I have not followed it 100%, but it has been a solid 90%. Since then I have had meat once (while I was visiting my dad, who my boys hadn't met yet and he cooked all day for us, so I ate the ribs) and I have had non-vegan items 3 times. So, I would say that is pretty good for a 5-month run (did ok when I was in Vegas but had some noodle stuff one night and threw it all up about an hour later).

With this diet that I am adopting now, I want to see if I can actually reverse the autoimmune diseases and combat the inflammation from the low back. I need to stick with it 100% and take out a few more items that are processed. Doing this for 50 days is going to also be an eye opener for me. I might have to cut out a few other whole food plant-based items. I know that I don't have a sensitivity to gluten, but I do have a sensitivity to corn and wheat. If I continue to eat those and I am still having flares, then I will adjust and take them out. We eat gluten free bread, which doesn't mean it is all amazing and great. Some are heavily processed and have the sugars that cause me to have flares and stuff, so I will be watching what is in those and buying the less processed brands. I am going to try to make my own bread as well. That just depends on if I have the energy to put into doing that. I have 2 bread machines, but it still takes energy. No more candy, no more shitty unhealthy chips and other things that are sweet and not good for me; and are probably causing some inflammation.

We have all seen the 250lbs vegans and wonder…WTF!!! HOW??? They can still eat shitty, just no meat and dairy. Cookies, chips, candy, cooking with heavy fatty oils…that shit doesn't make you skinny. So, I can always do better and that is the plan (not that I am 250 lbs. I don't need to lose the weight. I only sit at 150 lbs.). Those things are officially cut out and this is the beginning of the reversal.

Since I homeschool my youngest, my day starts with getting him up, ready, and settled in to start school. Luckily, we normally start at 9am, so we get to take our time and not stress or rush. Even though I woke up feeling a bit tired, from lack of sleep and a snoring husband who moves around… A LOT! I tend to not sleep so well. I have been averaging about 4 hours of interrupted sleep a night. Though I did get 2 hours of straight sleep and 6 altogether. I would call that a win. I started wearing ear plugs to help a couple weeks ago but failed to put them in until around 5am. I will say, since the ear plugs, I have been sleeping a bit better. With a better diet and ear plugs, who knows what kind of sleep I will be getting soon.

Started off a little rough, but it got better after I got some food in my belly and had my spark. My body was up and moving and I felt really good. Got some house stuff done. Read, researched, went to therapy, wrote, helped my son with his school, worked out, showered, went to *Target*, cooked dinner, cleaned the kitchen, got him in bed, settled down and wrote some more. Doing this much normally, I would have made it to: went to therapy, nap, rest, lay on couch, cereal for dinner. There was no way I would have had this much energy. Again, I think the dose change is helping, the little extra sleep that I was able to get, and it's too soon to tell if the diet has any affect.

Today was my first full blown day on my period (I had been on the pill for over a year, so I didn't have my periods). I jumped the gun and took ibuprofen to stop the cramping that I knew was gonna be happening soon. The cramps did start and then I waited all day to see if they were gonna come back. I have those cramps that come from the back and radiate to the front. Today the back pain was there, like my normal period stuff, but I didn't get any cramping in the front, well not any, it was so minimal that I decided to wait to take the next dose of Ibuprofen. The back pain went away and there are no cramps. Hmmmm. Makes me wonder, did being vegan make my period bearable? Since I have been "half assed" vegan, I have been on the birth control, so I haven't had a period since going vegan. So, this holds high hopes for me that I will be able to handle being a woman after all.

I totally forgot to have my after-dinner snack, so I must not have been hungry enough to have one. I will be trying to get up to 5-6 meals/snacks a day. This is day 1 so bear with me. Before, I would normally just have breakfast and dinner, so this plan will help me get better at eating in general.

I had some low back pain, but like I said above, that could mostly be pain from being a woman. I was able to walk through target without having to lean on the cart for support (but I was also in there for a shorter time than normal).

Joint pain from the Fibromyalgia I would say was a level 2. Which it is normally a 7 on days like this. I only felt the pain when I went outside though. My fibro symptoms do not tolerate the cold. Cold weather hurts so bad. I had a mild headache, but that only lasted for about an hour and went away on its own.

To help me with sleep tonight, I bought a foam pad to see if it will help make the bed a little softer and help it not be so painful on my body. I might have to use some CBD/THC to relax as well. It's almost 10:45pm right now and I feel like I have a ton of energy. I am trying to get on a sleep schedule. In bed at 11pm, put on some hypnotherapy and fall asleep by 11:30pm, but this is just wishful thinking.

Day 2: February 7, 2018

Food consumed

Breakfast: 2 pieces of peanut butter toast (store bought gluten free bread)

Snack: Strawberry banana smoothie (with rice milk, spoonful of almond butter and a handful of cashews)

Lunch: Edamame

Snack: Apple and almond butter

Dinner: 4 (small) gluten free corn tortillas with rice and beans tacos with avocado, lettuce, tomato, onion, vegan sour cream, sriracha, and lemon juice.

Beverages: Water= 68 fl. oz. Spark= 10 fl. oz.

Activity level

PT and then I took my youngest for a walk to try to gain some energy. That didn't work out the way I planned. I was even more exhausted when I got home, and it was only a 30 min walk.

I was active for 112 min and got in 7,026 steps

<u>***Medicine and Vitamins***</u>

The dose of hydro did not do its job today, but I need to stay on this dose for a while and see how I do. I did get a message on Instagram about taking Dexamethasone instead. It seems to have better results for people, so I will be looking into that and seeing if it will benefit me better.

(looked into Dexamethasone: Not for me).

<u>***Appointments***</u>

Today I had my Chiropractic appointment and Physical Therapy. These morning appointments are hard to get to, especially when I am so tired and stiff. The adjustment was a little rough because my low back was tight, but he does these amazing little massages that always feel good and I love the type of table they use. These are not "popping" adjustments like at every other chiropractor. They have a specific table they use, and it stretches the spine just a little to get some fluid and movement. He does some popping stuff and uses the clicker (I love my terms for everything).

PT was good. I liked the new routine the guy has me doing and even though my body was like "WTF are you trying to do when I am this tired," it felt pretty good and I was exhausted. We focused on hip flexors, glutes, and of course the core. Engaging the core is harder than it used to be, especially when done correctly. 40 min later, I had worked up a little bit of a sweat. For now, he doesn't want me to do any twisting and wants me to just focus on building a very strong core, strengthening the glutes, hamstrings, and low back muscles.

Energy and Symptoms

I did not sleep well last night. I actually don't know if I even slept. I was in that state of half-awake/half-asleep. I heard every little noise, and again…Didn't use my ear plugs. The CBD/THC did not help at all. I didn't feel a thing; my mind was still racing, and I was not relaxed.

I finally pulled myself out of bed around 8am, but then went and laid back down because everyone else was still sleeping. My son stayed in bed until 8:45am. For one night I would love to sleep like he does. I think my body would be able to do some major healing. I was hoping the padding would help, but I didn't really notice a difference in softness. I will be adding a second one on tonight to see if there is a noticeable difference.

Not being able to gain any energy, I decided it was time I listened to my body and ended up having to take a nap. Well, the nap didn't go great. I did put in the ear plugs this time and again, I was in the state of half-awake/half-asleep. When I did finally just get up, I felt ok. Still tired though.

I needed a pick me up because I was so exhausted, and I needed to get some fresh air, (when you are so used to running and being outside for exercise and then you are forced to do everything inside, that want to be out is something you should strive to get. Nothing beats being outside. Unless the weather sucks). I think from all the stuff I got done yesterday and the shitty sleep I got last night, today my body just said "nah. Not today." It was also chilly outside, and I didn't wear my hat. My ears got cold which then made my neck and shoulders ache really bad and the joints felt like they were defrosting. My whole body was in pain from being cold. I feel so old when I make these statements. It's like hearing your grandparents talk about how they can feel the change of weather in their bones. Yep, I can totally relate.

 Thankful I meal prepped and had some food I could just throw on a gluten free corn tortilla and call it dinner. The nice hot shower I have been thinking about all day is not gonna happen. The more I think about it the more my mind and body are in agreeance that it is not happening...and that is ok.

I did notice with having to eat 5-6 meal/snacks a day, that I am full all day. It is going to take my stomach a little time to adjust to eating so often. I had to force myself, so I won't be having an after-dinner snack tonight. But I am happy that I did eat 5 meal/snacks today.

Fibro Pain level today was about a 5. Achy all over and the feeling that my joints were defrosting, along with exhaustion. I felt pain in my lower back all day. It was that really annoying pain that just sits there all day, tapping you, but you try to ignore it when all you want to do its yell, "KNOCK IT THE FUCK OFF BEFORE I PUNCH YOU IN THE FACE", but you can't punch pain. All in all, today was not the best. You can't win them all.

Day 3: February 8, 2018

Food Consumed

<u>Breakfast:</u> Homemade hash browns (Air fryer- They were not that great. Need to figure out how to use that damn thing correctly).

<u>Snack:</u> Strawberry banana smoothie (Same recipe as yesterday- minus the cashews: ate the last of them yesterday).

<u>Lunch:</u> Totally skipped today. Got busy writing (because I also write other books and needed to finish to meet my deadline... Yay for procrastination. Boo for my tummy).

<u>Snack:</u> Homemade sweet potato chips (FUCKING YUM!!!)

<u>Dinner:</u> Seasoned tofu patty with mashed potatoes (that were instant. Don't judge- they only have 3 ingredients and they are still healthy AF).

<u>Snack:</u> 2 kiwis (which I ate right after dinner). Later in the evening- An apple with almond butter (yes. I eat this a lot because I love it).

<u>Beverages:</u> Water= 60 fl. oz. Spark= 10 fl. oz. Coconut Water= 8 fl. oz.

Activity Level

4 moves from PT. I was active for 71 minutes and got in 5,909 steps. I still call that a win.

Medicine and Vitamins

Got in my morning daily dose of Hydrocortisone and Fludrocortisone. I tell you what, I do not miss having to take all the other vitamins and crap. This makes my life a lot easier to swallow (get it haha). I missed my afternoon dose, because...I was writing, and I forget to, ok. Don't judge. I did take a double dose in the evening to make up for it though.

Energy and Symptoms

Another night of shitty sleep. I do not know what the deal is. I even smoked to get me stoned enough to fall asleep. It wasn't until I crawled into bed that I noticed.... I wasn't even buzzed. Not even relaxed, but I was in bed already and I didn't want to go back in the cold. I just listened to my book on Audible and didn't fall asleep. It took almost 2 hours.... How do I know? Because I had to restart the sleep timer on my phone three times (30 min timer). I tossed and turned and was up at 4:45am. Laying in bed; listening to my husband snore and wondering.... How many ways are there to smother someone in their sleep. So, in total I got almost 4 hours of sleep. Never good for a spoonie.

The only good thing about that was, my youngest was up at 6am. He came in the room a couple times and I sent him back to his. I was not ready to face the day yet. I was actually pain free laying in bed and he wasn't going to ruin that. I was relishing in this moment for as long as I could.

7am came and my body started to hurt, so I guess that was my "wake up" call. We got up and we had breakfast and started his school stuff. I was feeling pretty good; pain level was only at a 3 and I didn't feel tired. I had to take him to his speech therapy and since I can't stay for it, I went shopping. I had to pick up some groceries, so I could juice today. I do not normally shop at *Fred Meyer*, but it was right next to his appointment. Walking around felt ok. I was taking it slow and looking at all the fruits and veggies. I didn't realize there was such a thing as a purple carrot (grabbed that shit up). Got all my stuff for juicing and decided to grab a sweet potato and try to make some sweet potato chips.

When we got home I rushed to put everything away so I could sit down and finish the book I was writing. Just had to finish the last chapter. Forgot to eat, forgot to take my meds; but this needed to be done today. And it did.

When I got up from writing for 4 hours. Holy shit, my back was not happy at all. It was like someone stabbed me. So much pain and with each step it got worse. I had to juice, and I had to make those damn sweet potato chips. I was determined, and I was not going to let this pain bother me.

Juiced, which didn't take long but when you are in pain and you have to stand, 15 min felt like 3 hours. And then I was like, "Oh, I can still make the chips. This won't take long…. Famous last words. I didn't know what I was getting into. 2 hours later the chips were done. At this point my back was about a level 8 pain (the whole walking like grandpa in a walker pain). My legs felt like they were so swollen and that they were going to explode. My feet felt like I was walking on Legos.

I had to bring in a few pieces of wood for our fire place. When I walked down our stairs, my back froze, and I stood there for about 15 seconds. I couldn't even lift my leg. Those times it gets a little scary. Call me dramatic, but I often think "if I try to move at this point, will I become paralyzed?" That is how bad it scares me. No one should have to suffer from any kind of pain like this and have it thought of as nothing by medical professionals and disability.

When you are in this kind of pain so often, you have to do what you have to do. You deal with it and pray that you can get all the shit done so you can sit and rest. I still had to shower and I was not looking forward to that. I couldn't' go another day without a shower. I like to shower daily but missing 3 days wasn't gonna cut it for me. I let myself rest for 20 min and then hopped in for a quickie. When you go without for a few days, Lord have mercy; it feels so good. Thank God for my shower chair. You would think I was 80 years old. Listen… If you are in chronic pain and are a spoonie. Invest in a shower chair. You won't be sorry. It is the best thing.

Shower done. Now time for bed…. Crap. Wishful thinking. I have to write about my day. It's all good. I just took my laptop into my nice comfy bed and here I am.

So, all in all today was a shitty day. I was on my feet to much and paid the price for it. Oh, ya…. My legs and feet swelled up a bit too. Not to the point of explosion, but to the point of, "when did I gain 100 lbs." type of swollen. I guess you can't win them all.

Continuing on and looking forward to another day. It has to start getting better soon. Right?

Day 4: February 9, 2018

Food Consumed

<u>Breakfast:</u> 2 pieces of peanut butter toast (gluten free-store bought)

<u>Snack:</u> Strawberry banana smoothie (strawberries, bananas, almond butter, rice milk)

<u>Lunch:</u> Edamame

<u>Snack:</u> Apple and almond butter

<u>Dinner:</u> Tofu burger and baked beans

<u>Snack:</u> Pan popped popcorn (8pm) 2 Kiwi (830pm- to help with insomnia).

<u>Beverages:</u> Water= 80 fl. oz. Spark= 10 fl. oz. Coconut water= 8 fl. oz. Mean green= 4 fl. oz.

Activity Level

Got home and kept delaying my workout. I feel a lot better when I work out, even if it's just 20 min. My body needs the movement and if it doesn't get it, I have more of pain. It's like my body craves it. So, I finally did some PT moves (10 min) and got on the elliptical (35 min). I am realizing that I have been reading SO MUCH, that I am SO FAR behind on all my shows. Being on the elliptical in front of the TV helps with a better, longer, more entertaining workout. Motivation station right there. During the PT moves, I could tell my back was getting annoyed, so I made sure I was really engaging the core and taking that strain off the low back. Got on the elliptical and enjoyed some tv time. Felt really good. Nothing hurt, and I didn't feel worn down.

I was active for 97 min Walked 7,980 steps.

Medicine and Vitamins

I took all my meds on time today. You wouldn't think it would be so hard, but I tend to have my alarm go off to take them, and then.. Squirrel. I do take them…. Most of the time, it's just later than I normally would. Still not good.

Appointments

Went back to the Eye Dr. today because I went to the him last month for a new contact prescription and fitting. I found out a really interesting fact. The contacts he gave me to try didn't work out, so I was back to try a different pair. He checked my eyes again and then he asked me if I was diabetic. Because I have Addison's Disease, I have been borderline diabetic the whole time. He then told me that I should go have my blood sugar levels checked because people who are diabetic will have a change in their prescriptions. He didn't go into detail, and I didn't ask (if you really want to know; ask your eye doctor). So, he really stressed for me to get it check because I went from a 4.75 to a 5 (no clue what that means, but he thought it was enough to stress the blood sugar). So, my eyes will probably keep switching (which makes sense since some days I feel like I see better with my contacts than other days). I thought it was in my head, but now I know…. And so do you (at least a bit. You can always learn why and how on your own. I'm not that curious…yet).

Energy and Symptoms

Did the 2 kiwis last night to see how it would help with sleep. I was very skeptical about it, like I am about most things, but by 11pm, I was having a hard time keeping my eyes open. I was reading in bed, trying to finish the book, and it was a struggle. It took me about 10 min to fall asleep and then it was 7am and my son was waking me up. I felt like I slept hard. I haven't slept like that in…. I can't even remember. I don't even sleep that hard when I take 5 of my Doxepin and that will knock you out and make you feel like a zombie the next day (no bueno). I really felt that it worked, but I will be trying it out and see for the next week just how consistent it is and not just some placebo effect. Yes, I was skeptical, but it's still in my head.

I felt rested and was up with my son. Now, after getting out of bed, my back quickly reacted and was like, "Today I might just irritate you, just to irritate you," (Asshole). I did my best to ignore it and I used my core a lot of try to counteract the pain, and that really does help (when you remember to do it). I did good but could have done way better.

Another really annoying symptom I have, that also keeps me from working as a massage therapist, is that I have really shitty grip. I can't hold onto something for very long. That being said (and known by me), I tried to pick up a fire log. I normally carry it, with my palm up, for some reason, I was trying to grip it, palm down. Dropped it on the kitchen floor and it broke and got the little saw dust shit everywhere. Knowing I can't hold it like that, I deserved the mess.

Got dressed and went to my eye appointment. Dressed up a little bit, because for like the past month, I've looked like the troll under the bridge. Had on a cute pair of green skinny jeans with a cute darker green top and put on a yellow scarf. Ok, so it sounds like it didn't match, but it looked really cute. Went into the bathroom and grabbed the coconut oil, and then I touched my green pants…. So…. I have a cute pair of just regular, dark washed skinny jeans that replaced those. FUCK!!!! That better not stain. I put some dawn dish soap on it and will let that soak in.

When I got home, me and my husband talked about what we read in *How Not to Die*. It was just about the gluten and wheat stuff. If you haven't read this book, I highly suggest it. What we are going to do is, make our own bread and see if that affects us (mostly my youngest). There will be that slight change with this diet. There will be changes going on from time to time. This is 50 days of plant based, so I need to dive into all avenues. Even if it is putting gluten back in a bit and seeing how we react, or don't. And who doesn't like homemade bread. I control what is in it as well and we are looking for the least processed flour we can find.

On Friday's I pick up my friend's kids from school and visit with her after I drop them off to her. Always fun to sit and talk. Usually we sit at her dining room table and after a while my back will start to hurt really bad, but today it didn't, which was so great.

Got home and did my blog stuff, made dinner, and cleaned the kitchen. My little guy told me that he was going to help because they (him and his brothers) need to make it easier on me because I am sick and in pain all the time. Bless if little freaking heart. I love this kid. All the mommy feels.

Friday's are our movie nights, so we watched *Captain Underpants*. Just watching him watch it was entertaining. To him, it's the funniest thing ever. I was actually able to sit through the whole thing and watch it without having to move around a ton. My body would normally start to hurt so bad that I have to adjust how I am sitting like 500 times. Not today! I think engaging the core more and being aware really helped. So, I will have to keep that shit up.

Pain level was at about a 3. Minus the annoying back pain, that fluctuated throughout the day between a 2-5. No pain from when I was outside in the cold like I have been having and I had energy to make it through the day. Today is a win.

Day 5: February 10

Food Consumed

<u>**Breakfast:**</u> 2 Pieces of peanut butter toast (gluten free-store bought)

<u>**Snack:**</u> Strawberry banana smoothie (same recipe as yesterday)

<u>**Lunch:**</u> Edamame and mashed potatoes

<u>**Dinner:**</u> Medium french fries from McDonalds (My oldest had a game and we had to stop somewhere. They do not taste as good as I remember, and I have a feeling it will not sit well with my stomach)

<u>**Beverages:**</u> Water= 64 fl. oz. Spark= 10 fl. oz. Mean green (juicing)= 4 fl. oz.

(My meals are becoming so predictable. You should make it a game. "What did she eat toady?" And see how many times you can guess my meals correct. I promise it will become more interesting…. Or will it??).

Activity Level

Did some PT moves (only 14 min) and then got on the elliptical and watched some TV. I am telling you, TV helps and with the right shows, you can just go and go. I only went for 30 min, because I had shit to get done today (another basketball game that would require a 2-hour drive). Still a win for workout though.

I was active for 116 min and walked 8,823 steps.

<u>*Medicine and Vitamins*</u>

I missed my 4pm dose of Hydrocortisone but did take it at 5:45pm. I really need to stop skipping doses and take them on time. This is one thing that does annoy me about myself. I have the alarm on my phone, so it shouldn't be hard, but apparently, as soon as it goes off, I have A.D.D. I took 5 doxepin to knock me out tonight (I want to make sure I get healing from the driving and sitting).

<u>*Energy and Symptoms*</u>

Last night I slept good again. I got in 6 hours. I did toss and turn, but that was because I had baked beans (let me explain). The baked beans have brown sugar in them and brown sugar hates me and makes my body have flares. I got to go through that last night and it was painful. That is the fibro rearing its ugly head and saying, "you put brown sugar in your body and now we are going to punish you with horrible muscles pain that makes you feel like they are burning and will make you want to rip your skin off." ASSHOLE!!! It was not fun, but I am glad I was able to get 6 hours of sleep.

Had to be up early for my youngest son's basketball game. I hate that they play at 9am. No one wants to wake up early on a weekend, especially to watch 9 and 10-year-olds play. NO FUN!! I do love watching him, but I don't like that it's that early. He is tired still and not ready to play an hour worth of basketball. Sitting in the cold gym is not fun for the parents either.

I was doing ok from coming down from the flare but felt a little tired when we got home. I was debating on taking a nap or working out. Happy to say that working out won this debate.

Went to Target and got some bread to try and flour to make my own bread. I read through all the ingredients. I didn't realize how many brands put brown sugar in their breads. Those were a no go. After reading labels for 20 min, I found 2 that would work. I also looked through all the flours and picked one that just said flour. Didn't realize how much was in flour as well. I will be going to Whole Foods at some point to check out their selections.

My body felt better by the time we had to leave, but I was worried how it would be on the drive. I realized a while ago that the stadium pad I use for basketball games, works great for long car rides. Pushes my hips a little forward and takes the pressure off the low back (you should try it if you take long trips. It really helps).

I forgot to bring the pad into the gym with me, so I had to sit on the hard bleachers. It wasn't bad today. I was not in the pain I normally am from sitting on the hard bleachers. YAY!!! One thing though, my hands all the way up to my shoulders were really achy and starting to really hurt towards the end of the game…. From clapping to hard. Really??? Fucking clapping. Ya, thanks body. Thankfully though, that didn't last too much longer. It went away after about an hour.

I mentioned before that I had my oldest take dairy out of his diet for 30 days. This is day 5. His face is SO MUCH CLEARER. I was actually shocked at how much it cleared up in just 5 days. The redness has gone down, the inflammation, he didn't have all the zits that are always ready to pop. I would say his face cleared up about 60%. His girlfriend noticed and he kind of did. I had to point it out a little. So hopefully he will look in the mirror and go "Hey! It did clear up." I can't wait for him to notice when his sinuses start to clear. He doesn't like it because he says he can't have pizza. I will make him a pizza he will love that is dairy free, so he won't be all whiny about not having pizza. I don't blame him, pizza is amazing. I honestly like the vegan pizza we get, but I want to try this one recipe that just omits cheese and puts on a lot of yummy veggie toppings.

The drive home was good, no back pain with the drive. Got home and got ready for bed. The only thing that is hurting right now is the shoulders a bit, but not to bad. I would say today's pain level was at a 3 (and that was because of the clapping arm pain). The low back pain was about a 3 as well. I engaged my core a lot more today and I really think that is helping, so I am gonna keep being aware of that and do it ALL THE FUCKING TIME.

Because we were at the game, and there were only 2 places to eat. McDonalds or Dairy Queen. Which do you choose? I am sure the fries might haunt me later in the form of a flare, but hopefully I will be knocked out cold and wont' even notice. My kiwis aren't ripe, so I decided to take my doxepin (sleeping pills). I don't know what my body will feel like tomorrow from the driving and the game (stressful watching District Tournaments.... They lost by 1, so I was a little stressed). I want to make sure my body gets the good sleep, so I can heal. Better safe than sorry. Right!?!

Day 6: February 11, 2018

Food Consumed

Breakfast: 2 Pieces of toast with peanut butter (store bought-gluten free).

Snack: Apple and almond butter

Lunch: Multigrain tortilla chips and banana

Snack: Homemade sweet potato chips

Dinner: Leftover potato casserole from a few nights ago and edamame

Snack: Strawberry banana smoothie (rice milk, almond butter, almonds, and flaxseed).

Beverages: Water= 80 fl. oz. Mean green= 4 fl. oz.

Activity Level

I got on the elliptical for 30 min, got off and did 15 min of PT stuff and back on the elliptical for 15 min. Slayed it today!!

I was active for 107 min and got in 8,614 steps.

Medicine and Vitamins

I was late on all my meds today, but they were taken. When you read below, you will understand why there were each late.

Last night after I closed the computer and went to bed. I had the worst gas (sorry TMI-but this is all gonna be real. Like I said; the good, the bad, and the ugly). I am 100% sure it was from the McDonalds fries. Serves me right, should have gone with just the water and waited till I got home to eat. Gas isn't a bad thing, it's just not enjoyable.

As you read from yesterday, I took the doxepin to help me sleep, and oh boy did it help me sleep. I got almost 10 hours of sleep. I didn't wake up till 11:15am. I got up and took my meds (only 3 hours later than I should have…. oops), read for about 20 min and then went and laid down and took a nap for an hour and 15 min. Again, missing my meds and taking them and hour and a half later than I should have. I sat down and read some more and decided, since I need to meet my daily step goal, I should get off my ass and get on the elliptical. My mind was saying "sure, we can do this." My body was saying "Let's just go crawl back in bed and have another nap." My mind won, and I got my ass on that elliptical. I wanted to do extra, just to show myself that I could…. And I did!

My body was still saying "sleep," but I kept going. I got in the shower, did laundry, vacuumed the house, and cleaned the kitchen. Anything to keep my body from laying down and taking a nap. This just means I get to have an early bed time.

Ate the leftovers for dinner because I really didn't want to cook, and they needed to be eaten. I don't like to waste food, so it was a good call. Nothing wrong with using that as an excuse.

Today I am having a sweet tooth attack. I haven't indulged in it, plus we don't really have anything in the house that isn't WFPB compliant. I just want snickers and the green footie tootsie rolls and maybe some rolos. UGH!!! So glad we don't have candy in our house because it would all be gone right now. To curb the sweet tooth, I made myself a smoothie and that did the trick. So yummy.

Today's pain level was at a 1!!! How about that. Despite the side effect of the doxepin (exhaustion), I have felt really good. I was on top of engaging my core. There were only a couple times when I didn't, and I felt just a tiny pinch of pain and immediately corrected myself and engaged the core. I only had the slightest hint of pain in my hips and shoulders and that could be from laying around so much. I am thrilled that the pain was so low. I just wish the energy would have been up. I am really looking forward at how tomorrow is going to be. I feel each day gets better.

Day 7: February 12, 2018

Food Consumed

Breakfast: 2 pieces of peanut butter toast (What!?!?! SHOCKER!!-store bought gluten free).

Snack: Healthy mean green juicing concoction. (Yes, I can count this as a snack).

Lunch: Multigrain tortilla chips and edamame

Snack: Apple and almond butter (Did you guess correctly)?

Dinner: Rice and beans with sriracha

Snack: Strawberry banana smoothie (rice milk, almond butter, and flaxseed).

Beverages: Water= 80 fl. oz. Spark= 10 fl. oz. Mean green= 12 fl. oz.

Activity Level

It has been sunny the past few days and today I was not going to miss out on the opportunity to get some good Vitamin D. I let the sun soak into my skin while I enjoyed a walk at the track by my house. I made sure I bundled up good so my Fibro pain wouldn't mess up my fresh air. I got in a 30 min walk (the sun really makes you feel better). It's out and shining, begging me to come enjoy it; and I did. On the start of the walk I could feel my low back starting to act up. "Not today back, this is my day and I am going to enjoy my walk". I engaged my core and walked. That was hard, but it took the pressure off the low back and I was able to make it the 30 min. Plus, engaging my core is gonna give me super sexy abs, so I will not complain about that. Stretched a bit when I got home and everything felt good for the rest of the day.

I was active for 129 min and walked 9,124 steps. GO ME!!!

Medicine and Vitamins

I actually took everything on time today. I am slaying it. Maybe I can make this a habit. It could really help with my energy levels as well, if I could just be consistent with taking my meds on time.

Appointments

PT kicked my butt today. Love those balancing weight bars they have me use. I looked dumb and uncoordinated but felt the burn. PT guy (I honestly don't know his name) agreed it was time to kick my butt a little bit, so we did more with the centriforce bars. I am an athletic person, I have great balance, and I can do a lot of things, really good the first time. Except these damn bars. They really throw you off and I was so off balance. I felt clumsy; but I am also determined and stubborn. I corrected my mistakes and was able to make it look more like I knew what I was doing as opposed to a baby learning how to walk. BOOM!! Owned that bitch. It really fired those muscles in my low back and that felt great. Progress!! I always love getting adjusted. It really helps after having to go through PT first. Everything is warmed up and ready to be aligned.

I had another great night of sleep. Got in 6 and half hours. I was up at 7am, laid in bed for a while and got up to start my day. I was already feeling energized. My back was stiff but wasn't "hurting." Made myself some breakfast (shocker that it was peanut butter toast again). Got my son going for the day in school and got ready myself. Which never really happens if I don't have to be somewhere. Wasn't sure how long my energy would last, so I wanted to make the most of today.

I knew that I needed to meal prep, so I started with that. I got the beans and rice going. Peeled potatoes and cut them up and cooked them. Good breakfast option for me. (I am sure you are tired of seeing peanut butter toast, but I love eating it for breakfast. Try it, it's good). I also made a big pot of white rice for my little semi-picky eater. Got my blog page done before 9am. (Woot woot).

Continued on with my day as a stay-at-home mom. Finished up with my son's school, read, cleaned up a bit. Got ready for my Chiro and PT. Adjustments always feel good to me. There is just something about getting your body aligned that gives you those feel good vibes. I was glad that we stepped it up in PT today. He said I looked better and more energetic.

Rushed home and fed my youngest so we could get him to his basketball practice. 2 long hours of 9 and 10-year-olds practicing with a coach who doesn't care if they are listening to him. Tonight, all the kids were cranky AF. Attitude everywhere from everyone of them. Is it a full moon? Is it

National cranky kid's day? WTF. Did make for a more interesting practice though.

Driving home from his practice I was thinking about how this is my last year in my 30's and I would be turning 40 in June…. Wait? What? 35, 36, 37, 40…Really? Math skills on point. I'm just going to be turning 38. Where is my head? I tried to put the kitchen trash can in the fridge last week as well as trying to move a piece of wood that was in our fireplace (blazing hot with flames) with my bare hands. I am losing my shit. I don't know what my brain is doing, but it needs to focus. I don't want to go into a nursing home in my 30's. That shit can wait until I'm 90.

There was some stress today that I was trying to avoid (because being married isn't always sunshine and rainbows 24/7). I just took some deep breaths, let the hubby say what he needed to say and kept my mouth shut. Tried to move on from it, because I was not going to let it affect my day, stress me out, and cause an unnecessary flare. I actually thought about if for about 15 min and then let that shit go. I had other things I needed to think about and get done. Stress will not control my life and I am not going to sit and dwell on things that can't be dealt with in that moment. Life is a lot better when you don't sit and think, and rehash in your mind, and let it consume you. Give it a few mins and then move on. Affirmations come in handy here. I did notice that there was a cold sore forming at the end of the night (from the stess. Ugh).

As far as pain; the low back was at a level 1, then moved to 2 and ended with a 3. Engaging the core is helping and I did great for a big chunk of the day. Around 8pm is when it started to say "Ok. Let's get some rest before I really take this pain to a whole new level." I had only minor Fibro pain today and that was from driving in our van; that was blowing cold air and it was cold outside. Gotta get that taken in and looked at. I need my heat. But even with that, the fibro pain was at a 1 all day (3 with the cold). My energy level was great today. I got things done, didn't feel tired at all, made it through the whole day with some energy to spare. I am ready for bed now though. Sweet warmth and softness beckon me to crawl in and dream.

Day 8: February 13, 2018

Food Consumed

Breakfast: 2 pieces of 21 grain toast with peanut butter and potatoes (added a little something today).

Snack: Multigrain tortilla chips

Lunch: Cucumber/tomato salad and edamame

Snack: Peanuts

Dinner: Almonds (I can explain this)

Beverages: Water= 64 fl. oz. Spark= 10 fl. oz. Mean green= 8 fl. oz.

Activity Level

I didn't have time to get in a workout today, but I was active for 56 minutes and got in 4,337 steps

Medicine and Vitamins

I took my morning meds. I can't remember if I ended up taking my afternoon meds. I didn't want to double dose just in case, so I was going to take double in the late afternoon, but I ended up somehow missing that dose as well. I might be paying for this tomorrow.

<u>**Appointments**</u>

My weekly 'Bitch it out" session that I always look forward too. (aka Therapy!) Talked about how the diet is going, marriage, kids, people that drive me crazy and depression. Yes, depression comes with these lovely autoimmune diseases (don't pretend you don't have it. It's ok to admit). Just get the help needed and "grow" from there. Made some semi-major life decisions and hopefully I will get to share them with you all soon. We shall see how it all plays out, but everyone likes a good suspense; this is mine.

<u>***Energy and Symptoms***</u>

Woke up at 7am, ready to conquer the day. Had a lot of energy and a great outlook. I slept for 6 and half hours again, but I got a good 3 hours of straight uninterrupted sleep. HELLS TO THE YA! I knew today was going to be a pretty chill day, because of the driving I was going to have to do. Ate some breakfast, got my son going with school work, got ready for my therapy session. Oh, and woke up with no pain today. NONE. ZERO. ZILCH.

My oldest son has a basketball game that we are driving down for (2 ½ hours away), so I didn't want to have to sit for an extra 3 hours in traffic. We left at a great time because there was hardly traffic. When you suffer from back pain, the last thing you want to do is sit in the car for more than you need too. Fortunately, with this diet, I didn't have any pain; there or back.

Got to the game early and watched the team before my son's team play. I don't know what the hell is going on with these teens, but they are tucking their shorts up into their undershorts, or underwear and then rolling the tops (not all, but enough to make me notice). WHAT…THE…FUCK…. If they want to wear short shorts for basketball; get a time machine and go back to the 70s-80s. I do not understand this. Let's not make this a "thing" or "Fashion statement". JUST STOP IT! If your kids are doing it, slap them.

My son's team played great. OMG, my son had an amazing game, especially defensively. WOW! Proud mama; mama tears; screaming whoohoo mama. Unfortunately, they lost out. Bitter sweet ending to his Senior year. I'm sure gonna miss watching him play. Let's pray he gets a Basketball scholarship for college so I can continue to enjoy watching. During the game, my back did great. Only like a level 2 pain, but it was more of my ass that hurt sitting on those stupid hard bleachers then actual back pain. Going up the stairs didn't bother my back either. I was awful at engaging my core today, and guess what? I didn't have that much pain when I forgot. Just little tings here and there.

I missed dinner because of the game. You can't get a good plant-based meal at a high school basketball game, so I bought almonds. I was going to eat when I got home, but I am way to dizzy. I am actually sitting here typing; dizzy. Not so easy, but this needs to be done. I think that the stress for the game (they went into overtime and lost by 5-STRESSFUL) and missing my meds is what is causing this. Now that my body is winding down from that and the drive, it is starting to go "Ok, you need to do better at taking your meds, because at any time we can decide to just stop working for you and you will die." Not being dramatic, that is the truth.

My oldest told me tonight that he has to get his Senior project done and he has 2 weeks to do it. He is doing it on invisible diseases/autoimmune diseases. I love that he chose to do this so he can better understand what I have been going through the past 4 years. His face is looking even better and when I asked him if he noticed anything else, he said he knee hasn't been hurting for the past couple days. And all he is doing is not having dairy. Amazing!

With all of that being said, I had another great day. High energy, level 2 pain with the back. No fibro pain and just now with the dizziness from lack of taking my meds. It is almost 1am and my body has not failed me. You can't begin to understand what this diet has done for me and what it can do for you. I'm excited to continue and show you the results.

Day 9: February 14, 2014

Food Consumed

Breakfast: 2 pieces of 21 grain toast with peanut butter

Snack: Mean green

Lunch: Almond rice pilaf and multigrain tortilla chips

Snack: 1 piece of homemade bread

Dinner: Gluten free rotini spaghetti (the canned sauce was surprisingly really healthy)

Snack: Strawberry banana smoothie (same ole' recipe) and 2 kiwis

Beverages: Water= 80 fl. oz. Juicing= 8 fl. oz. Spark= 10 fl. oz.

Activity Level

Elliptical for 40 min and PT moves for 10 min. Turned on Netflix and watched some *Friends* while I used the elliptical. Today was the first time I did not have numbness. Usually my feet will start to go numb about 20 min into it and 30 min is usually my limit and I have to get off and walk around for a bit to get some blood flowing again. Today, I had very slight numbness. I always thought it was normal for being on an elliptical. I've heard other people talk about how that happens to them as well. Glad it is going away. Maybe I will be able to go a straight hour without any numbness. The past 2 times

I've been to PT, he has not sent me the exercises. I can't remember all of them, so I do what I can remember, which is only 5 moves. It would be nice to be able to go through the whole set.

I was active for 102 min and got in 8,640 steps.

Medicine and Vitamins

Took my meds all on time today. Have I even made it 2 days with taking them on time? Please, my Addisonians; take your meds on time. Don't be like me.

Energy and Symptoms

I went to bed around 2am. When I hit the pillow, I was ready for sleep. Though my sleep tracker said I tossed and turned a lot. I got 4 hours of sleep. I woke up at 7am ready to go. Got online and added some more books to my Amazon cart. Got up and blogged a bit and then planned out my day. As we all know, plans never turn out the way you want, especially when you think you can stay on a timeline.

Homeschooling my son, somedays, takes more of my attention than it should. By 3pm I got everything I wanted to get done, so I can't really complain. I was feeling a little stiff today. Really having to engage my core. The back pain today is very sharp and seems to be in a smaller, more focused, area than before (isolated to the Left IS joint-which is good-I think). I cleaned the kitchen, did 2 loads of laundry, grinded up some oats and flaxseed, and made 4 loaves of bread (well the bread machine did).

While I was taking a "reading break", I noticed that I was getting little chilly (wearing my workout clothes, because I still need to get that in), and my joints in my upper body were starting to feel some fibro pain (not bad, but I wasn't going to let it get out of hand). I moved over to the fireplace to warm up and it went away.

Towards the evening my back was acting up, just a tiny bit. Again, having to engage that core to help ease the pain. I had a ton of energy that lasted me through the day. It is now 9:15pm and I am starting to get sleepy (might be the kiwis).

Pain level today was averaging a level 2 (low back and the minor fibro pain I felt today). I am starting to feel that maybe I can get back in the work force. I still have another 41 days of this reboot to go, so we shall see how I do. If my grip would come back, I would definitely try again with massage. I really do miss my clients and helping people in general with aches and pains.

Since I didn't get to much sleep last night, I am going to go to bed a little bit earlier and hopefully get some good rest tonight.

Day 10: February 15, 2018

Food Consumed

Breakfast: Cubed potatoes

Snack: 2 pieces of 21 oat toast with peanut butter (switched it up).

Lunch: Almond rice pilaf and edamame

Snack: (Skipped)

Dinner: Vegan homemade pizza (flour/oatmeal dough)

Snack: Strawberry banana smoothie (rice milk, almond butter, and almonds)

Beverages: Water= 64 fl. oz. Spark= 10 fl. oz. Mean green= 16 fl. oz.

Activity Level

55 min of PT and it was tough. I was active for 121 min and got in 5,815 steps.

Medicine and Vitamins

I took all my meds on time today. I dropped my morning dose down to 2 Hydrocortisone, so we shall see how I do with getting through the day with energy and fatigue. I will give this a week and if I start to feel like I am starting to struggle I will adjust it back to what has been working for me. I have a feeling that I won't need to. This reset has been pretty amazing.

Appointments

I was so happy to go to my PT and Chiro appointment. I knew something was off, and I just couldn't pinpoint it exactly. PT guy (I should probably learn his name) and I discovered that it was my SI joint. It must not have liked me sleeping on my back. We did some work to help release it and kicked up the intensity of the session, then I went and got adjusted; focusing on the little fucker. Doing some of the PT moves made it radiate all the way to my shoulder. Thank you, rotators and multifidi (little muscles that run along the spine).

Energy and Symptoms

I only got 5 hours of sleep last night and woke up (or should I say was woken up) at 6am. Apparently, I slept on my back all night. Fell asleep on my back and that was how I woke up. I know I moved around because my sleep tracker said I did, and I think I remember getting up and going to the bathroom. I never sleep on my back. I guess I was snoring pretty loud too.

I wish I could have gone back to sleep, but my youngest thought it was a great time to be awake. Usually he is good on his own and I can go back to sleep, but for some reason he needed the extra attention this morning. Since I was up, I made the most of it. Instead of my usual PB toast, I made myself some potatoes. I fried them up (using broth instead of oil). Made my son some toast and started him with school work at 7:30am. He got 1 problem in math done and was complaining that he was tired. Really child? You have to pick your battles and I knew that if I sent him back to bed with no tv, he would be coming back to me in about 10 min. I was wrong. He fell back asleep until 9:15am. I wish I could have crawled back into bed, but I had consumed a spark and I knew that wasn't going to happen.

This stupid fucking cold sore on my face is so huge, red, and disgusting looking. It hurts so bad and doesn't seem to be getting better. It was all crusted over and bleeding (graphic, I know). So gross. I hated that I had to leave the house with this grotesque sore on my face.

By 10:30 am, I was so hyper. I had so much energy (thanks to the spark). I made homemade pizza dough, got some editing done, read a bit, helped my son with his school. I had all the energy, but my back was bothering me. Hindering a lot of what I wanted to do.... Like going for a long walk outside. Even when I engaged my core, it was still a little painful. But it was isolated to my left side to one very tiny spot (that mofo SI joint).

I came home and moved 60 fire logs from the car to the house. I stabilized my core and only carried a few at a time. I was sore for a couple hours after; from my appointment and moving the fire logs, but the SI joint was feeling a lot better. Not going to sleep on my back tonight. The only reason I did was because of the monstrosity on my face. I avoided going grocery shopping today because the cold sore is so bad. I am hoping it is better tomorrow because we really need some food. I ran out of my mean green juice, so I need to get more veggies, so I can make some more.

The only pain I had today was that SI joint stuff. I didn't even have Fibro pain going out in the cold. The back pain wasn't all that bad, only about a level 3. I am really happy with all the results I am getting and I'm hopeful I will be back to running soon.

It is 10pm and I am ready to crawl into bed. It's been so great to have "normal" days. Get up, have energy to make it through the day and get shit done, and by 9:30pm-10pm be ready to meet the sandman.

Day 11: February 16, 2018

Food Consumed

Breakfast: Peanut butter toast (21 oat bread)

Snack: Potatoes and 2 pieces of toast (No butter)

Lunch: Breakfast blend (fruits I juiced)

Snack: Apple and almond butter

Dinner: Rice with steamed broccoli and carrots

Snack: (none)

Beverages: Water= 80 fl. oz. Spark= 10 fl. oz. Breakfast blend= 8 fl. oz.

Activity Level

I turned on a movie and got on the elliptical and then did PT moves. I was only on the elliptical for 45 min, did some of my PT stuff for 20 min, then got back on the elliptical for 15 min. I was sweating so bad and it felt amazing. Jumped in the shower and let the hot water relax and soothe my muscles.

I was active for 127 min and got in 10,363 steps.

Medicine and Vitamins

I was only late taking my afternoon meds by 45 min. I was distracted by all the stuff I was getting done today and forgot. My attention span is not great. I should just start letting my alarm continue to go off until I actually take the meds.

Energy and Symptoms

I slept great last night. I got 6 hours of sleep and was up at 7am. I got up and had breakfast and went and sat back in bed and read a book until 8:30am. What a great way to start my morning. After I got out of bed to deal with my youngest sons constant nagging to play the computer, I made him make his own breakfast as punishment. I know…I am the worst mom ever.

I was a little hungry again around 9am, so I made myself some cubed potatoes with toast. Since I am taking oils out of my diet (not completely, just using them as little as possible). I wasn't sure how I would like dry toast, but it was fine. I didn't miss having butter on it.

My cold sore is looking a bit better and not hurting as bad, so I decided it was going to be ok to be seen in public. I went to Whole Foods and got a bunch of fruits and veggies for juicing and meal prep and then some other groceries. The cashier was talking to me about the food I was buying, and I told her the cliff notes version of my story and she was amazed. She said her son has an autoimmune disease and is on a ton of meds and he wants off. I suggested that she have him read _Food over Medicine_ and try to go whole food plant based. She was pretty excited, and it felt good to share my story, brief as it was. That really got me even more excited about this journey and how I get to share it with all of you "spoonies."

Got home and started everything. I made homemade pasta sauce and juiced a fruit breakfast blend and a mean green. I was on my feet juicing and cooking for 2 ½ hours. My back was hurting, but only at a level 5 pain. My feet were doing good. Which normally they would have been in a lot of pain. I sat down and rested for 15 min and I was good to go again.

Finished up with the pasta sauce (turned out so good) and then started making dinner. I used the rice cooker to make a huge batch to have for meals this week. I was on my feet and moving so much today and had all the energy to make it, but I did realize that I would not be able to work in a job where I had to be on my feet for more than 2 ½ hours. Any longer and my body would be screaming at me. I miss working so much, but until I can get this all under control and I know what my limits are, I am stuck at home, testing my limits and learning...and healing.

My older boys came up this weekend. My oldest sons face looks amazing. He said one of his friends even gave him a compliment about how much his face has cleared up. We started talking about other things he has noticed, and he said that when he was at his girlfriends, helping with loading hay, he didn't sneeze at all. He said he usually sneezes the whole time, but he didn't. 11 days in. He is starting to get better with accepting the no dairy lifestyle. He is still bitter about the pizza and not having mayo on his sandwiches, but there are other options that he will discover. He is also doing his Senior project this weekend about Autoimmune/invisible diseases. I am happy that I get to help him and be one of the people he interviews. He was telling me about some of the things he learned and stories he read. I love that he is gaining knowledge and wanting to understand what I have been going through. I have the best boys EVER!!!

The only pain that I had today was from being on my feet for so long, but after resting it was fine. My rest/recovery time was amazing. Usually it's a day. Today, it was 15 min. I look forward to crawling into my bed and sleeping so my body can fully recover. I pushed it pretty good today and it deserves some rest.

Day 12: February 17, 2018

Food Consumed

Breakfast: Breakfast blend

Snack: Breakfast blend

Lunch: Mean green

Snack: Mean green

Dinner: Gluten free pasta and homemade pasta sauce with homemade french bread

Beverages: Water=64 fl. oz. Breakfast blend= 36 fl. oz. Mean green= 36 fl. oz.

Activity Level

I was only active for 52 min and got in 4,316 steps (slow day).

Medicine and Vitamins

I took my afternoon meds a little early because I had a massage that cut into the time to take them. All my others were taken on time. I am getting a little better at remembering.

I had a massage today. The girl was pretty good. She is from Dublin and had an amazing accent, so of course I kept her talking. I really needed that massage. I wish I could get 2 a month, but 1 is better than none. I might have to move that up to more a month, because I know my body really needs it.

Energy and Symptoms

Slept pretty good last night and woke up at 7am. For some reason my youngest and middle son were up at that time playing video games. They were not being very quiet, so I decided to finish reading 2 of the books I was almost done with. I am at 31 books for this year already and its only February 17th. I woke myself up a little more and started getting ready for the day. I wanted to juice all day (give my body a little reset) and then have dinner. I still had the energy to get me through my day. I might do the same thing tomorrow.

I spent 3 hours helping my oldest write his Senior Project Report. He had already been working on it for 2 hours when I joined in. We knocked out a huge chunk of it and will finish it off tomorrow. This kid and his procrastination. Wonder where he gets it from........???

For dinner I did homemade French bread. OMG!!! So amazing. It was a big hit with the boys. The pasta sauce turned out good, but I know that I need to add more herbs to it next time. They smelled really potent when I put them in and I didn't want to overdo it, but I underdid it. It wasn't bad, it was pretty good, but could be better.

I wasn't very active today because I was helping my son with his report. I did notice that my eyes were not focusing like they should. From learning about the blood sugar and eye connection from my ophthalmologist, I wondered if my blood sugar was off a bit. Having just the juices could do that.

Pain wise, I was really good. The back felt good, no fibro pain. I did go to best buy and was walking around looking at laptops, and I had to sit down finally when we were getting ready to purchase one (which still hasn't happened. I have to wait until Tuesday). My back started to hurt a bit, so I didn't want to push it.

I am definitely ready for bed now. It is 11:23pm and I feel that I pushed my brain to the limit today. I am actually starting to feel a little dizzy right now, so I think its time to go give my body a good night's rest.

Day 13: February 18

Food Consumed

<u>Breakfast:</u> Homemade oatmeal bread with peanut butter

<u>Snack:</u> Breakfast blend

<u>Lunch:</u> Edamame

<u>Snack:</u> Banana

<u>Dinner:</u> 5 corn soft tacos (beans and rice, refried beans, avocado, salsa, vegan sour cream, and sriracha)

<u>Snack:</u> Strawberry banana smoothie (fresh ground almond butter, rice milk, handful of almonds) and 2 kiwis.

<u>Beverages:</u> Water= 80 fl. oz. Breakfast blend= 16 fl. oz.

Activity Level

I got in a really good workout while the boys and my husband played their video games. I got on the elliptical for 40 min and then did my PT moves for 20 min. I am really having a hard time holding back on my workouts now that I am feeling better. I really want to push myself, but I am waiting for my chiro to release me to do more. I don't want to rush into something. My body is starting to crave running more, I just have to be patient.

I was active for 129 min and got in 10,784 steps. Killed it!

<u>*Medicine and Vitamins*</u>

Took all my meds on time today. Now if I can just be consistent with this, it will make my body a lot happier.

<u>*Energy and Symptoms*</u>

For some reason last night, I was pretty gassy. I assume it was from drinking the juice all day. It wasn't painful, just annoying. I slept pretty good too; about 6 hours. Tossed a bit but woke up feeling well rested. I slept in until 7:45am and was the first one up. I sat and read in silence for an hour. The boys finally got up and quickly made their way to the video games.

I had a lot of cleaning I wanted to get done today and decided that I would delegate. I don't ever do this, so it was nice not having to clean the whole house by myself. I didn't even have to ask the kids twice. I just told them what chores they would do today, and they got up and got them done. SO NICE!!!

I still have the grotesque sore on my face. This is the longest I have ever had a cold sore. It is just not wanting to go away. It's so embarrassing that it has lasted this long. JUST GO AWAY!

Helped my oldest finish off his Senior Report. I think he did a great job and can't wait to read the finished paper. Got lots of reading in today, 3 chapters done on my book edit, made homemade chocolate chip cookies, and played *Cards Against Humanity* with the boys. Such a weird game to play with your teenagers. Awkward moments, but it was a blast.

My youngest was so cranky this evening. Everything bothered him, he didn't want to eat his dinner and cried like 10 times about nothing. I am so glad he went to bed early. He needs about 12 hours of sleep to reset himself.

I am tired; today wore me out. I was up and moving around and had my brain going more than normal. I like that it's 9:15pm and I am ready to crawl into bed. My body didn't hurt today from any fibro pain. I had lots of energy again and made it through the day great. I woke up with my back feeling like it was slightly bruised. I made sure I engaged my core for everything I did today, and it kept the pain level at 2 when I was bending and doing house stuff. The rest of the day, when I wasn't being as active, I didn't have pain at all. NO PAIN!!!! Do you know what that means? My body is healing. I have had some fluctuation with pain, mostly in my back, but this is HUGE. I am on my way to having an active "normal" life and that feels pretty damn good.

Day 14: February 19, 2018

Food Consumed

Breakfast: Cubed potatoes and 2 pieces of homemade oatmeal bread

Snack: Breakfast blend

Lunch: Edamame and mean green

Snack: Apple and almond butter

Dinner: Leftovers (4 tacos)

Snack: Banana, 2 kiwis, and breakfast blend

Beverages: Water= 80 fl. oz. Spark= 10 fl. oz. Breakfast blend= 24 fl. oz. Mean green= 24 fl. oz.

Activity Level

Did PT for 36 min at the office and when I got home I really wasn't feeling like doing any other workout. I just wanted to knock out more of my book edit and relax before the week starts (today was Presidents Day, so everyone was off school). I dragged my ass onto the elliptical and picked a movie to watch. I only did 30 min, but with PT and that, I felt it was enough. Some days you feel it and some days you don't, but you just do it…. You won't be sorry.

I was active for 112 min and got in 6,692 steps.

Medicine and Vitamins

Yay me!! I took all my meds on time again. I hope I can keep this up. It shouldn't be hard to remember to take pills, but I am human and make mistakes…. Unfortunately forgetting to take meds that help keep you alive is not something you want to forget.

Appointments

I realized that I didn't have any pain this morning. When I first got up, I was a little stiff, but it went away after moving around for 10 min, but other than that, there was no pain. I was so happy to tell my PT and Chiro this. I was hoping that this would sway them into letting me start working out harder. No such luck. My chiro wants me to just keep doing what I am doing until the full 4 weeks are up and then we can look out how I am and slowly start to add things in. I am ok with this. I fully trust his judgement and expertise.

Energy and Symptoms

I slept really good last night. I got 6 ½ hours and I got a good 2 ½ hour chunk of straight sleep. I was up at 7am (I like this early morning thing). Everyone else was asleep so I slipped into my writing room and read for 2 hours. It was so peaceful and quiet. I almost forgot what it was like to read in silence; without being interrupted. Once my youngest was up, I made him some breakfast and then set him up to play some video games so I could knock out a big chunk of my book edit. After that was done, I laid in my living room where the sun was shining in and read for an hour.

Today was moving fast, but I was enjoying the peacefulness of it. I made us some lunch and then I started getting ready for my Chiro and PT appointment. At this time, I was thinking about how the day had gone and how I was feeling. I didn't have any pain. WOW!!!

Relaxed for the rest of the evening and read my book. When my little guy went to bed, I knocked out some more of the book edit. Today was great. I can't even express how excited I was having a day with no pain (some minor low back fatigue with PT). I feel that my mood is better as well. I am not grumpy and irritated at everything. I actually look forward to doing things. My energy wasn't as high as it has been, but I was also reading a lot today and just keeping it low key, so I didn't really test the energy level.

There is one thing I want to adjust. I have noticed that I have been bloated. I haven't really addressed it, but I was thinking today that I shouldn't have any bloating. So, for a week I am going to eliminate wheat all together (I'm going to miss having it so much). I want to see if that is what is causing the bloating, which sadly, I have a feeling that wheat is the culprit. This is going to be really hard, but I know I can do it and it will be worth knowing. That way I can adjust and only have it 1-2 times a week, instead of 3-4 times a day.

It is time to turn in and sleep like a baby (hopefully).

Day 15: February 20, 2018

Food Consumed

Breakfast: Banana and breakfast blend

Snack: Mean green

Lunch: Edamame

Snack: Apple with almond butter

Dinner: Bowl of rice with tamari sauce

Snack: 2 kiwis and strawberry banana smoothie (rice milk, almond butter, almonds, and flaxseed).

Beverages: Water= 64 fl. oz. Breakfast blend= 16 fl. oz. Mean green= 16 fl. oz.

Activity Level

No workout today. Active for 42 min and got in 3,566 steps.

Medicine and Vitamins

I was only 30 min late in taking my afternoon medication. Not good, but not too bad. If I had them strapped to my arm in a little "pill bracelet," I wonder if that would make it easier for me to remember to be on time.

Energy and Symptoms

I think I slept ok last night. It says I got almost 5 ½ hours, but for some reason it showed a gap in sleep (as if my tracker was off my wrist). I don't know what happened there, but I know I didn't take it off around 5am. So, I am thinking that 40 min gap, I must have been asleep. I did sleep until 7:54am. I also didn't fall asleep until almost 1am. My mind was going crazy. I thought I was tired until I laid down and then my brain was like "let's look on Amazon at all the things we want to buy." I couldn't stop looking at stuff.

Once I was up, I made my youngest some breakfast, and quickly remembered that I am cutting out bread for a week to see about the bloating thing. I really wanted peanut butter toast on homemade bread. I settled for a banana and some breakfast blend.

 My son had speech therapy today, so I sat in the parking lot and read for a bit. I made sure I parked my car so the sun was shining on me the whole time. It was nice and warm. It's been really cold outside and I didn't want to keep the car running for an hour. Plus, vitamin D is amazing when it's natural.

My husband started to get sick yesterday, so I quarantined him to the writing room (we have a futon in there). I didn't want his nastiness all over the house and with me not having much of an immune system, I can't have him out and about. I wish we had the money where he could just go stay at a hotel until he was better. Wouldn't that be nice to do, just go stay in a hotel while you are sick.

I went to best buy to get my new computer. OMG!! I am in love with it so far. I got the *HP Envy* touchscreen. I was nervous setting it up because I wasn't sure if I could remember all of the things that would need to go on it and I didn't want to spend all day loading and trying to figure all that stuff out. To my surprise, when I was going through the initial stuff with the Microsoft password and the computer booting up, the picture I had as a screensaver on my old computer popped up on this one. Boom!! I didn't have to do anything. Everything was already on there, plus all my bookmarks were saved from the internet. This computer stole my heart.

Got some editing done and set up a WFPB plan with a friend of mine so she can start getting on the right track to help with her arthritis and back pain. I am excited for her to start this journey and get to feeling better. It will also help me to see if health coaching is something I can do. I have the energy now to do things, and I want to work from home so that I am not overstressing my body and disappointing employers. I have to be realistic with having Addison's disease. I still have limitations. I will see how it works for her and how much work I will be putting into keeping her on track and getting her through her first 30 days. I have another friend who wants to try it out as well, so adding her into the mix will help me see what I can take on.

I was disappointed that I didn't make time to workout. I didn't come close to my active goal or step goal. I will just have to be ok with that and kick ass tomorrow. I did meal prep this evening though, so I'm still a badass. With the meal prep done, it will be easier to stay away from bread. Though tonight, after I ate dinner and had a smoothie, my stomach is bloated. I did have a bowl of rice for dinner and that is a grain. One thing at a time though.

My back was a bit stiff today. It stayed at about a level 2 pain all day. I had lots of energy and no fibro pain. The back pain was just annoying and constant. Being on my feet to meal prep, wasn't too bad. It did make the pain jump up, but only to a 4. I sat down when I would start to feel it tighten up. It's very helpful being aware of that now. Engaging the core still and just trying to listen to how my body is handling it. After having no pain yesterday and a level 2 today, I know that I am not ready to run or push my workouts yet. My chiro knows what he is talking about. Wishful thinking on my part to think that 1 day of no pain would mean no pain from here on out.

I am doing so much better than before and I can't explain how amazing the results have been for my life. I am only 15 days into this, so not even halfway and the results that I have had speak volumes for WFPB lifestyle and how it can help with pain. I am not saying that it is reversed... Yet. But I am on my way there.

Day 16: February 21, 2018

Food Consumed

Breakfast: Hash browns with onions and spinach

Snack: Skipped-totally forgot because I was juicing

Lunch: Edamame, brown rice and quinoa with brussels sprouts and carrots

Snack: Mean green

Dinner: Brown rice and quinoa with potato/brussels sprout/asparagus/spinach casserole

Snack: 2 kiwis

Beverages: Water= 80 fl. oz. Spark= 10 fl. oz. Mean green= 8 fl. oz.

Activity Level

37 min of PT at their office and 30 min on the elliptical. I was hoping that the elliptical and tv would help relieve some of the stress from today, but that was a bust.

I was active for 116 min and got in 6,791 steps.

Medicine and Vitamins

I did all my meds on time today. Woot woot! I feel that I should get an award for this. It's not as easy as it seems.

Appointments

When I got to the chiro he adjusted me and I felt pretty good, but when PT hit and we started going through some exercises, my back was like "FUCK NO!" It started to hurt and stiffen up. I had to lay there for a while and he did some stretches on me. I love when people stretch me out. If you haven't had it done, you should. (Thai massage is great for that, if you are wondering). I was able to make it through, but my back jumped from a 2 to a 4.

Energy and Symptoms

I was up at 7:20am this morning. I laid in bed until about 7:45am, checking my phone and looking at Pinterest. I slept for 6 hours and 40 min. I am getting so close to that 7-hour mark. Maybe it will happen tonight.

I was up and getting ready because I had an early appointment today. I made myself some hash browns with spinach and onions in it (super tasty). My back was feeling a bit stiff this morning, but I was hoping it would go away after moving around for a bit.

I had to go get some veggies at the store, so I was not looking forward to walking around with my back acting up after my appointment. It did ok though. It settled down and allowed me to walk around with minimal pain.

I got home and juiced, which was probably not the best idea. My pain jumped from a 2 to a 5. I sat and rested for a while and the rest of the day it stayed at a steady 3 with some sharp pains here and there. I was very diligent about engaging my core though. It has been so cold the last 2 days, but I didn't have any of the fibro pain when I was out in it this morning.

When I got home I started my son with his school work, this is where the day went to shit. He fought and fought and cried and bitched and moaned and threw fits and cried some more. 5 hours to do 3 pages of math (2 of the pages only had 5 problems on them). The stress he was causing me was giving me heart palpitations, I was starting to feel the numbness in my face (I get numbness when I know I am stressing to much). I was trying to not let him affect me, but he was hell bent on having his way (which I am not sure what that was). He got his electronics taken away, he got bedtime tv taken away, and he got his *Beyblades* taken away. Didn't seem to phase him until he finished with his school work (at about 5pm). He realized everything he had lost and he had nothing to do…. But complain. He has so many toys, but it wasn't enough. I had Pandora radio going on the computer and he sat and stared at it.

I got on the treadmill to help me de-stress, but it didn't work. This child just wouldn't let up. He was trying to plead with me. He wanted me to take away electronics for 2 days, so he could play with his *Beyblades* today. I stuck to my guns and told him no.

Finally, bed time came, and he wanted me to read to him. Which I don't mind doing. I grabbed a book and thought this would be nice. I started to read, and he started to poke my arm. I pushed his hand away and told him to stop. Did he? Nope. He poked me again and I pushed his hand away. He poked me again and I told him, if he didn't stop messing around I would not read to him. Did he stop? NOPE! He started to blow on me. Sorry kiddo, you blew it again (haha... see what I did there). I told him that I was done, and he could go to sleep. I left his room and turned off his light and told him goodnight. He cried for 15 min. Overdramatic sobs.

I needed to do some breathing to help calm myself. I let him cry it out while I got the rest of my stuff done for the night. He came out and asked for a second chance and I told him he already used up his second chances, but he could turn on his light and read on his own. I am really surprised that he did. I swear he better be good tomorrow or he won't live to see another day. Having a child on the spectrum is rough. You want to be a little more understanding of what they are going through, but I also want him to understand that he has to suffer the consequences of his actions. It is really hard lesson for him to learn, but hoping that one day it will just click.

I was able to get a little bit done. I got more of my book edit done, juiced, and posted on my blog. I had so much more I wanted to do today, but that went to shit. My body will not be able to handle any more stress tomorrow.

I have a friend who got in touch with me who wants to end her fibro pain, so I will be talking with her tomorrow and setting her up on a plan. Maybe this is something I can do and help people discover how much better they can feel on the WFPB plan. It is exciting. I was thinking about all these years I have been in so much pain and how my health declined. I wish I could have found this sooner, then I wouldn't have had to miss out on so much, but can't dwell on the shoulda, woulda, couldas. I am doing it now and that is what matters.

No fibro pain today, fluctuating back pain between a 2-5. I would call today an "ok" day. Could have been better, but I will take it. Still had some bloating, so I am curious to what could be causing it. I still need time for the wheat to leave my system. It might be all grains and I'll have to give up rice and quinoa as well. Could be a certain vegetable, which would be a lot harder to track down, but this is a process and I will figure it out. I still have a lot of days to go.

Day 17: February 22, 2018

Food Consumed

Breakfast: Hash browns with onions

Snack: Mean green

Lunch: ½ avocado, rice, and edamame

Snack: ½ apple with almond butter

Dinner: Brown rice and quinoa with brussels sprouts and carrots

Snack: Strawberry banana smoothie (rice milk, almond butter, and flaxseed) and 2 kiwis

Beverages: Water= 80 fl. oz. Mean green= 10 fl. oz.

Activity Level

Nothing to exciting today. I just did PT moves for 25 min and got on the elliptical for 30 min while I watched some T.V.

I was active for 108 min and got in 8,057 steps.

Medicine and Vitamins

Took all my meds on time again. Gotta make it a habit. I notice that I have been doing really good when I am consistent in taking my meds (who knew).

I decided I was going to sleep on my back last night to see how it would affect me since yesterday wasn't the best day for pain. I felt that I slept great, but my sleep tracker says otherwise. I did have more upper back pain, but my low back felt amazing. When I got up, it wasn't stiff. I was able to move around really well. It didn't start to hurt until about 5pm and even then, it was only up to a level 2. I am going to try to sleep on my back again and see how it feels tomorrow. If it does good, then I am going to go back to my side and see if there is a difference. I think I can deal with the upper back pain way better than I can deal with the lower back pain.

This morning it was so nice to have time to myself. I read by the fireplace while the house was silent (I can get use to mornings like this). I also had time to finish my book edit. Yay me! I sent it off to the beta readers, so now I just have to wait for them to get done.

My son did so much better today. I don't think my body could have handled another day like yesterday. I would have lost my shit. It went smooth and he was a joy.

I got my friend set up with her WFPB plan. I am excited for her because she suffers from Fibromyalgia as well. She eats healthy too (except she eats way too much cheese), but I can't wait to see how she does with a better plan. It has done so much for me, I just can't wait to see how it affects my friends. I love too see people get back to a better life.

Today was such a beautiful day and I should have taken advantage of it, but I just had random things to do that prevented any outside time. I hate days like that. It's not that I had important things to do, it was just things that consumed my day that really shouldn't. I am hoping I will be able to take advantage of the weather tomorrow… That is if it is as nice as it was today. It was cold, but the sun was shining bright.

My oldest son got his acceptance letter from WSU. I am so proud of him and all the hard work he has put into his high school career. He was accepted to WSU Vancouver a couple months ago, now this one is for Pullman. I selfishly want him close to home, but I know I must let him spread his wings. He will be 18 soon and I just can't deal with it. They are supposed to stay young forever until we are ready to let them go, but I am not ready. It's to soon.

I didn't have bloating all day…. That is until I drank the smoothie. I started to bloat 30 min after I finished it. I will see how my stomach is tomorrow. It would be great if it was the smoothies that made me bloated and not bread. I can give up smoothies way easier.

Today was really uneventful. But I was thrilled to pretty much have no back pain. No fibro pain either. I went outside in the cold and it didn't hurt my body. I know that it hasn't been hurting it lately, but I am still in shock at how I am feeling. I had great energy today, but it did diminish around 7pm. I was definitely ready for bed. It's 9:05pm right now and I am working hard to keep my eyes open. My youngest is still awake, so I can't go to sleep until he is out. These are days when tranquilizers should be legal to use on your kids.

Day 18: February 23, 2018

Food Consumed

Breakfast: Banana and mean green

Snack: Mean green

Lunch: Brown rice and quinoa and edamame

Snack: None

Dinner: 5 tacos (corn tortilla, brown rice, quinoa, beans, avocado, sriracha, and vegan sour cream)

Snack: Homemade chocolate chip cookies

Beverages: Water= 70 fl. oz. Spark= 10 fl. oz. Juicing= 16 fl. oz.

Activity Level

I got in an early workout. I turned on a movie and just went to town. I spent 45 min on the elliptical and did about 15 min of PT moves. My workouts have been feeling so routine, that I am getting bored with them, but today I felt like it was good. Might have been the movie I was watching, but I didn't feel like I wanted to quit, but I do need to start mixing it up. After this next week I should be able to start doing more and that will hopefully give me the motivation I need.

I was active for 110 min and got in 9,112 steps

<u>*Medicine and Vitamins*</u>

Another day of taking all my meds on time. I am on a roll. Feeling good and having a ton of energy.

<u>*Energy and Symptoms*</u>

I woke up a couple times last night, but I stayed on my back for most of the night. I had to lie on my side because it was hurting my upper back so bad, but my lower back felt great. I also got 7 hours and 20 min of sleep. I got in some really good chunks of sleep too. I woke up at 7:15am. My youngest woke up at 7:30am and he still looked tired, so I told him to go lay back down. He fell back asleep really fast and slept until 9:15am. I had 2 hours of quiet reading time by the fire. It's been so nice to have these days and I hope they continue. It is a great way to start the day.

Last night after I had the smoothie bloating, I wanted to see if it could be the banana that was causing the bloating. I ate a banana for breakfast and had some bloating. Sucks, because I love bananas. I just won't have them often, but alone, it didn't cause as much bloating as it did with all the other smoothie ingredients. The bloating went away fairly quickly too.

I went to go get my friends kids from school and I got pulled over. I wasn't doing anything wrong, so I thought it might be a tail light out. I was still shaking a bit and could feel my face starting to go numb. I guess that stressed me out even though I knew I didn't do anything wrong. He asked me for my license and registration. I didn't have a current insurance card with me (which is weird because I always put them in right when we get them) and he told me that our tabs were expired (They expired February 15th so it's not like it was a month or more). We never got a letter about our tabs and the officer told me that for the most part they don't send out anything letting you know. How the heck are people supposed to know? It's one time a year and who pays that much attention to their tabs? This could have been a VERY expensive ticket, but I didn't get one. He was cute, and I flirted a bit, nothing obvious or gross, just some womanly charm. I am glad he pulled me over though because I would have NEVER known the tabs were expired. I was surprised at how much it affected me (Addison's disease wise). My face felt numb, my chest got heavy, I got a little blurred vision, headache and dizzy. I had to sit for a couple mins after he left to calm myself a bit. Addison's disease always rears its ugly head unexpectedly.

Glad to say the rest of my day was boring. I didn't need any more "excitement."

I wanted to try wheat again, since I knew the smoothie was the culprit to my bloating. So, I ate the corn tortillas. So far (2 1/2 hours later), I have not had any bloating. I will have homemade bread tomorrow and see how I do. I did make chocolate chips cookies and ate one. I totally forgot I had put brown sugar in them (I make the dough and freeze it and cut it up, so I can just place and bake). It was so good. OMG, it's been so long since I've had a chocolate chip cookie. Not my best idea. I am having a flare right now. It's only been 2 hours and my body is not happy. It's not as bad as it has been in the past, but not fun. I will have to figure out a substitute for brown sugar and see how they taste. This flare is about a level 6 pain (brown sugar usually sends me to an 8, so I guess that is a plus). Was the cookie worth it? NOPE. It was good, but flares are no fun. All my joints feel like they are on fire and every move I make hurts. Even typing is hurting, but I am pushing through the pain.

I am happy to say that I didn't have any back pain today, so that was good. I wonder if my abs will start showing soon since I have to engage my core so much?

Day 19: February 24, 2018

Food Consumed

<u>Breakfast:</u> 1-piece homemade oatmeal toast with peanut butter

<u>Snack:</u> none

<u>Lunch:</u> Avocado on homemade oatmeal toast with sriracha and edamame

<u>Snack:</u> Apple with almond butter (I think I need to pick another snack)

<u>Dinner:</u> Sushi- Rainbow roll and Da Bomb roll

<u>Snack:</u> none

<u>Beverages:</u> Water= 80 fl. oz.

Activity Level

Got home around 7:30pm and I didn't want to waste a day not exercising, so I just did 30 min on the elliptical (I hardly broke a sweat, but I wanted to at least move my body some).

I was active for 94 min and got in 8,436 steps.

Medicine and Vitamins

Got them all done and on time. I think I might have needed to stress dose today. If I have any type of flares, I think it would be wise just to do that to help my body recover correctly. Stress dosing is a tricky thing, and you never really know when a "good time" would be to do that (unless it's obvious, of course).

<u>Energy and Symptoms</u>

I was in so much pain last night I didn't think I would be able to sleep. I did finally fall asleep and slept for 4 hours and 40 min. Even with that little bit of sleep, I felt pretty rested this morning. I was up a 6am and couldn't fall back asleep. I stayed in bed trying until 7am and then decided to get up and have another peaceful morning of reading. I am telling you, if you love to read and can wake up before your family, it is the best way to start the day.

I was still in a little pain from eating the cookie, but it wasn't too bad. My youngest had a basketball game early this morning, and by the time that was over, the pain had gone away. We got home and had some lunch and then I just felt like being lazy. I did get some things done, but I wasn't gonna try to do too much since I had a rough night.

I read almost all afternoon and then we headed over to a friend's house to hang out. It was nice to just sit and watch a movie and eat sushi. I do let myself have that treat, but after the last 2 times that I have had it, I think it will be easy to give up. Meat, though it be seafood, just doesn't taste as good anymore. I can easily live without it. A few hours later my stomach wasn't feeling so great. A little nauseous, so I think it won't be worth having again.

I did not have any back pain today, which was so nice. There were times when I would move and I could feel it starting to react, but I quickly engaged my core a little more, just to let it know "I got you boo," and then I was able to finish off the movement. 2 days with no back pain has been amazing. The residual fibro pain sucked, but it wasn't bad. It was a great day, albeit pretty boring, but I think we need those "boring" days sometimes.

Day 20: February 25, 2018

Food Consumed

Breakfast: 2 pieces of homemade oatmeal toast with peanut butter

Snack: None

Lunch: None (I don't even know how I skipped this)

Snack: None

Dinner: Chips and Salsa and a LTA (Lettuce, tomato, avocado, sandwich- went to restaurant)

Snack: Coconut chocolate ice cream

Beverages: Water= 80 fl. oz. Spark= 10 fl. oz.

Activity Level

I got on the elliptical (40 min), turned on the T.V. and enjoyed my workout. I really wanted to do more, but this was all the time I had, and was lucky enough to get it in.

I was active for 106 min and got in 9,618 steps.

Medicine and Vitamins

Another day of getting all my meds taken on time!! Should I stand up and give a speech? "I would like to thank my alarm, for always letting me know when it is time to take my meds. Also, to my brain. Though you have failed me many times, I have to give you props for giving me so many days of remembering."

And…. Moving on.

Energy and Symptoms

My stomach started to hurt after I got into bed last night. I was feeling a little nauseous but was able to fall asleep. I slept for only 5 ½ hours, but it was good. I woke up at 6am and struggled to fall back asleep, so I got out of bed at 7am and read. I started reading *The Female Brain* last night because me and my friends were going to watch the movie tonight together and I wanted to get the book done. I really liked both movie and book (highly recommend).

I am making a habit out of taking the mornings to myself and I do not regret it. My house was cold this morning, so I don't know if it was the cold or a residual affect from the sushi, but I had a slight flare this morning. I think it might have been the sushi since the cold hasn't really been bothering me lately. The flare only lasted until around 3pm and it was only about a level 4 pain, but still enough for me to be 100% sure that I am done with all sushi.

My son slept until 10am, so I got in a good 3 hours of reading. I should have made myself breakfast or tea, but I was pushing to get the book read. Once he was up I got him going for the day and went back to finishing the book. I had some teasers to make up and some writing to do as well. The day flew by so fast.

I did a quick workout, showered, and got ready for my friend's birthday party. This would be my first time going out to a restaurant (that wasn't a sushi place), so I was a little nervous about what they would have for me to eat. I ended up getting the Nachos, but having to take everything off, It ended up just being chips and salsa. I also ordered the BLAT with no bacon and no mayo. It was really good and I can make this sandwich at home.

It was so great to get out with the girls and laugh and talk. We watched the movie and it was one that would could talk about after, and since I read the book, I could dive into more of the science that was talked about in the book and not the movie. This lead to great discussions and how, we as mom's and wives, need to stop catering so much to our kids and husbands and really make some time for ourselves so that we can de-stress and relax and just enjoy quiet alone time. My friend had mentioned that her son gets mad when she goes into the bathroom to do her business. She is with him all day long and that little bit of time is nice, but when he is telling her she can't go or is in there with her, it isn't "relaxing." My other friend, whose kids try to make her feel bad because she works, and they say she doesn't spend enough time with them, when she really does (just not in their little kid minds). We have to have our own time when we are not bombarded with kid stuff and wife duties. This is why they have the show *Snapped*. We can lose our shit pretty quickly, so let us have our moment of peace. Sadly, mom nights end early, especially on Sundays and when kids have school the next day, but it was a great few hours that we did get.

When I got home, I saw that not everything had been done (except video games being played) that needed to be, so I finished up the last load of laundry in the dryer, emptied the dishwasher, and cleaned up the kitchen…Things that I should not have to do at 10:30pm, but I did because I was too pissed to just leave it. I was trying not too stress about it, but I knew if I left it, my stress and anger would be more dramatic than if I did it and just cursed under my breath about it. It is done now and that is all that matters.

Ladies, I can't stress this enough: HAVE "YOU" TIME! Make yourself a priority. When you have kids and a husband and a chronic illness, you really have to make sure you are ok. Whatever you can do to find that time, please do. We are the glue, so we have to be strong.

Day 21: February 26, 2018

Food Consumed

Breakfast: 1 ¾ pieces of homemade oatmeal bread with peanut butter

Snack: Banana

Lunch: Edamame, brown rice and quinoa with avocado, ½ piece homemade garlic bread

Snack: Multigrain tortilla chips

Dinner: 1 piece of homemade oatmeal toast with peanut butter

Snack: none (had dinner at 10:20pm)

Beverages: Water= 90 fl. oz. Spark= 10 fl. oz.

Activity Level

My youngest had his last basketball practice tonight. They had the parents involved in the whole 2 hours. I was nervous about how my back would do and I didn't want to overdo it, but I am way to competitive to not give it my all. I was really shocked that my back held up. It got up to about a level 3 pain towards the very end. I was amazed at how good I still am at basketball and I had a blast. My son told me "I could tell because of your smile. Who could miss that big smile, you were so happy." Be still my heart, you are the sweetest little thing ever. He kept checking on me during practice. He came over with my water to make sure I was drinking during one of the drills and then when we would take water breaks he kept asking me how my body was doing. OMG!!! This is kid. If you don't have a son like mine, you totally need one. He loves taking care of me and wants to make sure that I am always ok.

I was active for 175 min and got in 10,701 steps.

Medicine and Vitamins

I took my morning and afternoon meds on time. I had PT that interfered with my late afternoon one and my sons' basketball practice messed up my last one (and I was on a roll).

Appointments

I went to my PT appointment and I was doing really good, until he made me do child pose. Trying to get up from that was extremely painful. My low back is still hating to have to do those types of stretches. It didn't take me as long to come out of it, but long enough that I know I am still not ready for low back stretches. My chiro has now released me for fast paced walking on the track and down to 1 time a week to see him. We are both thrilled with the progress and just hope that my back will continue to get stronger.

Energy and Symptoms

Last night was a shitty sleep night for the most part. Even though I'm benefiting from sleeping on my back, it is killing my upper back. I put a pillow under my shoulder and turned my head in the opposite direction to help with the pain, and it did somewhat. I slept for 6 hours, but it didn't feel like I slept well. I was up at 6am again but was able to fall back asleep. I slept until 8am (I haven't done that in a while). I got up and had my peace and quiet reading time. My youngest got up at about 9:30am but was still tired so he decided to go back to bed and he slept until 11am. He came out pretty upset at me because I was making too much noise in the kitchen. I have shit to do child. You can't just sleep and expect me to wait around silently. Get your ass up! I think he might be going through a growth spurt, because he is sleeping in a lot. Though, last night he was up past midnight.

I meal prepped today and was able to stay up on my feet with no back pain this time. I was moving around a lot and not standing still as much, but it was great to be able to get it all done and not have pain.

When we got home from basketball practice, getting out of the car and walking inside was a bit rough. My back was hating me. After driving home, it got a chance to cool down a bit and the muscles were not happy. I grabbed an ice pack and laid on my dining room floor and just relaxed for 15 min. Got up and ran myself a hot bath with Epsom salt and baking soda, sat in that for 15 min, and now as I am sitting here writing (I have the ice pack on my back right now and my bed warmer is on high just waiting for me to come and settle for the night). My hips are a bit sore as well, they haven't moved like that in a very long time. I really hope I will be able to walk tomorrow.

Today was such a good day and this will help me see what my limitations are. Though I was only released to do fast paced walking…. Basketball practice might have been a bad idea. I haven't been able to play with my kids in YEARS and with me feeling as good as I have been, I was not going to miss this opportunity. I have already missed too many things.

My eating was off today because of the times that my appointments fell and my sons practice. I will do better tomorrow. Right now, it is time for me to go relax in my nice warm comfy bed and try to heal.

Day 22: February 27, 2018

Food Consumed

Breakfast: Hash browns with onions and 1 piece of homemade oatmeal toast

Snack: Mean green

Lunch: Edamame

Snack: Apple and almond butter

Dinner: Homemade pizza with vegan cheese and vegan sour cream (for dipping)

Snack: none

Beverages: Water= 64 fl. oz. Mean green= 12 fl. oz. Spark= 10 fl. oz.

Activity Level

No workout today. Maybe tomorrow. I was active for 45 min and got in 3,895 steps.

Medicine and Vitamins

All my meds were taken on time today. Going to really try to stay on top of this again. I can't have multiple days of missing meds, really messes with my energy levels.

I propped myself up slightly last night to see if it would help with the shoulder pain. It worked! I slept hard last night. I got 7 hours and in that 7 hours, only 37 minutes of it was light sleep. I slept until 7:40am too. I did wake up in the middle of the night to use the bathroom, and holy shit, my foot and knee were killing me. I limped my way there and back. My back felt GREAT though. I couldn't believe it. Unfortunately, it was ruined by foot and knee pain. When I got out of bed to go read, I decided to ice my back, just to give it that extra little love. I also iced my knee and my foot. The foot bothered me all day, the knee pain only lasted until mid-day, and only hurts when I touched it. It feels like it is bruised, but there is no bruise there.

I was going to cancel my Therapy session but decided to keep it and I could hobble myself there. I had my husband drop me off while he took our son to speech therapy. I brought a book to read, since I was 15 min early. I got caught up in reading until I realized I had been reading for a long time. I looked at my watch and it was 10:54. My appointment started at 10:45 and she was NEVER late. I pulled out my phone and checked my email. She sent me one at 8:45am that she was sick and wouldn't be in. SO WEIRD!! I checked my email at 9am and again at 10am. I didn't see it. I found it funny that I was going to cancel, and then it ended up she did. It was a day that I had my husband drop me off instead of driving myself, go figure. Did this stress me out? No. I was also reading the book *The life-changing magic of not giving a fuck*. So, that was a "fuck" I was not giving.

My son struggled with school today. I knew he was not feeling that well. His eyes were a little glossed over he looked like he could hardly keep them open. He was overly emotional. We made it through school (ending at 5:30pm). I gave him silverbiotics, immune booster, mean green, and some melatonin, rubbed his feet and chest with Vicks Vapor rub and essential oils going in the diffuser. He has a big day tomorrow and I don't want him to miss out. He is really looking forward to it and I am looking forward to a day to myself. Early bed time for this little guy and hopefully lots of rest.

I didn't have much of an appetite today and it felt like a slow day. I didn't want to do a workout, not that I really could because my foot hurt like a son of a bitch. I took today as a light day and really didn't do shit. Tomorrow I will totally kill it though.

There was no fibro pain today and the back pain was about a level 1. It was just slightly sore from having to jump while shooting. I am hopeful that it will do amazing on my walk and soon I will be back to running. Maybe this summer I can do another half marathon. I am so jealous of my middle son who is doing one this weekend. I wish!

I look forward to going to bed so I can wake up and have a day to myself. Every mom's dream come true.

Day 23: February 28, 2018

Food Consumed

Breakfast: Hash browns and 1 piece of homemade toast

Snack: Mean green

Lunch: 5 tacos (corn tortilla with rice and beans, vegan sour cream, and sriracha)

Snack: Apple and almond butter

Dinner: Edamame and strawberry coconut yogurt

Snack: none

Beverages: Water= 80 fl. oz. Mean green= 10 fl. oz. Spark= 10 fl. oz.

Activity Level

Did some PT moves for about 20 min and then went on a walk/run around the track (walked the corners, jogged the straight away). I wanted to test out how my body would handle a little running. I am still feeling sore from Monday, but in a good way. The back isn't in pain, my foot hurts, but not so much that it would stop me, and my knee is all better. My hip is a little sore, but that was from digging into it with the tennis ball. I put on layers and headed to the track. I was a little nervous to run but reminded myself that I was able to do basketball practice for 2 hours, this was going to be way easier.

I love running and I didn't want to stop on just the straight away. I wanted to push myself… But I was smart, and I didn't. I don't want to do too much too soon. I will take this week to see how I react to a little bit of jogging. I stayed out there for 37 min and enjoyed it. It was chilly and I should have layered up my bottom half, but I was happy to not have any fibro pain from the run.

I was active for 90 min and got in 7,791 steps.

Medicine and Vitamins

All meds were taken on time. WHOOP WHOOP!! I know it's only 2 days in a row, but I am taking that as a win. I have to encourage myself and celebrate the little things.

Energy and Symptoms

Last night before I got into bed I got out the tennis ball and started rolling it around the right shoulder that is still bothering me. OMG it felt so good. I also did my low back and hips. Rolling on a tennis ball is not something you want others around for. Some of the movements are a little…. Embarrassing to do in front of others and let's not forget the sounds you make because it hurts so good. I was thankful no one was there to see or hear me. After crawling in bed, I read for a bit until my son was passed out. I knew that he would not sleep great and that would mean less sleep for me. I kept my ear plugs out, because as a mom, we are the only ones who hear the kids get up. Which I do not mind taking care of my littles when they are sick. I think moms should because, to tell the truth, we do a hell-of-a-lot better job (the moms who are good anyways ▯). I was right. Sleep was really shitty last night and it wasn't just because of my son. I was thinking about how he was feeling and worrying that he wasn't going to get any sleep and every little sound was waking me up.

He got up at 3:45am and sounded so much better. He was even ready to go for the day. I was not letting that happen, so I gave him another round of last nights remedies and sent him back to bed. He woke up at 7:45am and told me that what I did worked. He still had a little stuffy nose, but he was full of energy. This child was crazy energetic this morning. He was talking 100mpm and excited over everything. So glad he was leaving with his dad today. It is their "gotcha" anniversary. Every year (for the past 7 years) they go out and spend the day doing "Father/son" stuff. That means I got the day to myself. I needed it because I was exhausted.

After my workout at the track, I went home and stretched it out, ate some lunch, and took a nice hot shower. When I was in there, I turned the faucet so the water would get hot and for some reason it kept getting cold…. Wrong way dummy. UGH!! Gotta love those moments.

After my shower, I decided, since my body was feeling a little exhausted today, I would take a nap. It was only about a 20 min nap, but it was just what my body needed.

The husband and child came home earlier than I expected but, little guy was starting to get hit with exhaustion and the hubby didn't want him to get sicker, so they came home so he wouldn't get worse (which is smart, but I was enjoying my time alone).

While they played video games, I went and finished reading, yet another book. And then headed out to Whole Foods with a friend to help her get on track with the WFPB plan. I love going there, it is never busy and it's not overwhelming. Tonight, it smelled like cigarette smoke over by the deli section, which was weird. It was like someone was smoking in the store.

Got home and I am ready for bed. Today I just felt run down. Nothing like it was before, but I think I could have easily slept all day and still have gone to bed and slept fine. I was semi-productive and that was good for me. My body right now is telling me to crawl in bed and rest, so that is what I am going to do.

Day 24: March 1, 2018

Food Consumed

Breakfast: 2 pieces of homemade bread with peanut butter

Snack: none (side tracked by the sun)

Lunch: Edamame and 3 tacos (rice and beans, avocado, sriracha)

Snack: Black bean chips and pico de gallo

Dinner: 2 pieces of peanut butter toast (because I am lazy sometimes)

Snack: Coconut butter pecan ice cream

Beverages: Water= 100 fl. oz. Spark= 10 fl. oz.

Activity Level

I decided to go walk/jog the track again. The sun was shining, and I wanted to take advantage of that. I bundled up, because let's be honest, it's still cold as a mofo; sun or not. I got in a great workout (walked 3 laps for a warm up: Walked 100m, jogged 100m x3: Walked 200m jogged 200m x3: Lunges 50m, walked 300m, lunges 50m: Finished with walking 2 laps-46 min). After my lunges though, I could really feel it in my legs. The middle of my cool down, I felt like my legs were going to give out. I walked home, but it was slow and by the grace of God that I made it without falling. When I got home and collapsed on the floor. I did 15 min of PT and then started to stretch it out, hoping it would help and stayed on the ground for a while to give my legs a break. When I got up to finally get in the shower, my legs said "nope, sit your ass down in a nice hot bath." So, I listened.

I was active for 112 min and got in 10,324 steps.

Medicine and Vitamins

ALL…..ON…..TIME!!!!!! The one thing about Hydrocortisone is that it only lasts a few hours, so missing doses, really messes with that level of energy you need to make it through the day. I will be excited when I do remember to take the meds. I am not happy though when my body is so exhausted, I take the meds on time, but I still have no energy… Life as an Addisonian sucks.

Energy and Symptoms

I slept pretty decent last night. I had my ear plugs in because I knew my little guy was feeling better and that he would sleep through the night. I got 6 hours and 43 min of great sleep. I have been sleeping in the past few days, but I think it is because my body is trying to recover from Monday's 2-hour basketball extravaganza, and yesterdays little "shock to the body" workout, and then today's workout and oh ya…. Aunt flow stopped by. So, my body is just trying to "heal."

Aunt flow came 2 days early, which was kind of a surprise to me since I didn't have any cramps. I am only spotting. As the day went on I got the mildest of cramps. Barley enough to notice. Ginger and WFPB is not joke when it says it helps with cramps and period flow. I couldn't be happier because the hell that my period was before would take me down for 3 days. HALLELUJAH!!!

After I got out of the bath, I had just enough energy to get to my bed. Rested and read for 45 min. Finally, my body was like "ok, we are tired, but we will let you get some shit done… So, don't take advantage of it."

I listened and sat down and started the new book (until my husband had to leave for work), helped my son out with the rest of his school work (so I sat there next to him-mostly playing on my phone), got a hold of a few friends and asked them to help me write my "mom" book, and then when I felt my body was ready to get some things done, I did all the things I wanted to do (made some homemade bread; in the bread maker, and threw in a big pan of brussels sprouts, carrots and spinach for some light meal prep). It wasn't a lot of things, but it was the two main things I wanted to get done.

I am taking it easy for the rest of the night. My son is in bed and I am gonna finish up last minute bedtime stuff and sleep like a husband or teenager…. Because babies wake up too much during the night.

Day 25: March 2, 2018

Food Consumed

<u>Breakfast:</u> 2 pieces of homemade toast with peanut butter

<u>Snack:</u> none (late breakfast)

<u>Lunch:</u> Edamame with a bowl of brown rice and quinoa, brussels spouts, carrots, and spinach

<u>Snack:</u> Multigrain tortilla chips with Pico de gallo

<u>Dinner:</u> 4 tacos (rice and beans, pico de gallo, and sriracha)

<u>Snack:</u> 2 homemade chocolate chip cookies (made with coconut sugar instead of brown sugar)

<u>Beverages:</u> Water= 70 fl. oz. Spark= 10 fl. oz.

Activity Level

Got on the elliptical for 50 min and watched some TV while I sweated my ass off. Did some PT at their office for 25 min (He talked way too much today and had me doing some stretches…. And lots of sitting and listening to him talk).

I was active for 132 min and got in 10,072 steps.

Medicine and Vitamins

Like a boss!! All on time.

Went to my PT appointment and the guy would not stop talking about random shit. I was super annoyed because I sat there for most of it. Though my legs were sore from the lunges yesterday, he did have me roll them out. Yes, I whined like a little bitch. It hurt so bad and not in the feel-good way (legit, had tears in my eyes), but I know it was good for me…. Right?!?! Once that was done, I got adjusted, and to me that always feels amazing. He told me to take it easy this weekend and let my body recover a bit. I can go for a walk, but no jogging until Monday. I think I can manage that. (Please oh God let it rain all weekend so I am not tempted).

Energy and Symptoms

I slept so hard last night. I got a huge chunk of sleep (almost 3 ½ hours straight-which is great for me). I got a total of 6 ½ hours and woke up feeling good. I was awake at 7am, so looks like my body has made a good recovery and is wanting to get back into the routine it was loving. Instead of doing some reading today, I checked my emails, made some teasers for my books and then checked some social media. Very productive morning.

After I got my son going for school, my plan was to get some meal prep done and some writing, but he had a different plan for me. He decided he was going to struggle with doing math again. This time instead of giving in, I let him fail on his own. I gave him 50 min to get it done and he got 3 problems done. He got electronics taken away. I sat down next to him and pointed to each problem saying "What is that?" Let's just say he HATED me repeating that over and over, but he finished 3 pages (minus the 3 problems he did on his own) in 15 min. Insane. He knows it, but just doesn't want to do it. I can't stress about it, because that's not good, so I just make him (because, yes, I am that mom).

Once that was over, he was on a roll and finished his other work quickly and without fuss. Which was great for me because I was able to get a bunch of shit done and started my new book…. I am sure you moms will LOVE!!

Talked to my oldest today. He said he has noticed that he hasn't had any allergies, not even around the horses and hay!! He said his face is about the same, still clearing but way better than it was. Recovery time from sports is still faster than it was before, which is awesome. His runny nose that was always a constant annoyance (I think more to me than him) has gotten a lot better and today was the only day it wasn't even bad. His allergies are FINALLY getting better. I'm not gonna lie, he is a heavy breather (think of the kid from *Hey Arnold* that was always breathing around Helga-for those of you old enough to know the show). It's going to be nice to not have to sit next to that, because you kind of want to punch him for it (even though it's not his fault).

I was talking to a friend about doing meal prepping for a "side job" and helping people with their diets. I love to meal prep and if I can change someone's health or chronic disease for the better, than I will do what I can to help them. It's just talk, but we shall see where it goes. I already feel like I have so many projects going and life happening, but I do want to help people and make a difference.

I made chocolate chip cookies today and instead of brown sugar I used coconut sugar (the dark stuff because it resembled brown sugar). I was worried about how they would turn out, but OMFG!!! Best cookies that have every graced my lips. They were perfection. Now I wait and see if they affect me. Part of me hopes so because I would eat those every day for every meal (thank God I have self-control). So far, I am feeling fine, which is fantastic.

My flow (sorry TMI) was a little heavier today (not by much, but it was there), but no cramps. Now I just wait and see if it lasts the usual 7 days or if it will be nice a short.

The only pain I have had today was the little bit in my left foot (still trying to recover), the soreness from the lunges, and about a level 1 in the back. Only certain moves would send a sharp shooting pain, but it only lasted for a second. The rest of my body was just workout sore. Which is good. I had a little more energy today and I feel like I will be back to my new improved WFPB body by tomorrow. I think another night of good sleep is the little boost I need to get there.

Day 26: March 3, 2018

Food Consumed

Breakfast: 2 Pieces of homemade toast

Snack: none (at my son's basketball game)

Lunch: Edamame and 3 tacos (rice and beans, pico de gallo and sriracha)

Snack: Apple and almond butter

Dinner: Pasta with homemade sauce and 2 pieces of homemade garlic bread

Snack: 2 homemade chocolate chip cookies

Beverages: Water= 80 fl. oz. Spark= 10 fl. oz.

Activity Level

It was so nice out and I wanted to get in steps goal met, so I took my son on a walk. The sun was out, but it was really chilly. We got too cold and just kept the walk to a mile. All that vitamin D was awesome, but it was too cold to stay out more than we did. He wanted to jog every time we hit a shadow. It was nice to do some jogging with him. When we got home I did 20 min on the elliptical.

I was active for 110 min and got in 10,186 steps.

Booyah!! All meds on time!! I was hoping to see an improvement in my energy levels with having all my meds being taken on time. Getting the right dosages at the right times is really hard. People who have working adrenal glands, don't ever have to worry about the times. Their adrenals just pump what they need, when they need. I have to take meds at times that I think my adrenals would produce cortisol. Super frustrating. 4 years... You think I would have this figured out by now.

Slept for 6 hours and 10 min. But I struggled all night. Woke up at 8am and laid in bed and read. It was so nice and cozy warm in my bed, so I didn't want to leave it.

My littlest had his last basketball game today (so thankful the season is over and we can have a little break before the next sports start). He wants to do swimming next, my middle one is doing track and my oldest is doing baseball. SO MANY SPORTS!!

I was really exhausted and struggled a bit today. I needed a pick me up (and by pick me up I mean nap-but that didn't happen). After my son's game I took him to get some shoes. This child's feet grow so fast. He is only 9 and is in a size 7 ½ - 8. I wear an 8 ½ - 9. WHY DO THEY HAVE TO GROW SO FAST?!?!?! He isn't that picky with his shoes, so it is always really quick.

When we got back I got some house stuff done, thinking the whole time, *I should go and nap while he plays the computer.* Instead I cleaned up a bit and then we went for a walk.

My middle guy ran his first half marathon today. He said he underestimated how far it was. I told him a week ago that he needed to train for it. I can't wait to run in a "race" with him this summer (if I am able to run that far by then). I want to sign us up for a 10k to start. I am not sure I will be able to do a half marathon anytime soon.

I am so exhausted and ready for bed. I took 2 doxepin tonight to help me get some sleep. I had no pain, besides that 3rd day soreness from my track workout on Thursday. Glad to say there was no flare from the chocolate chip cookies. YAY!!!

Here's to a good night's sleep. I think my body is still struggling to heal. Realizing I still have some limitations, but I am thrilled it is just exhaustion and not pain and fatigue.

Day 27: March 4, 2018

Food Consumed

Breakfast: 1 Piece of homemade toast with peanut butter

Snack: none (didn't get out of bed until 10am)

Lunch: Edamame and rice with brussels sprouts and carrots

Snack: 1 homemade chocolate chip cookie (BTW, still good even when they are not fresh out of the oven)

Dinner: 4 tacos (rice and beans, avocado, pico de gallo, and sriracha)

Snack: 2 chocolate chip cookies (fresh out of the oven)

Beverages: Water= 84 fl. oz. Spark= 20 fl. oz.

Activity Level

I did 15 min of PT moves and then I got on the elliptical (even though I didn't want too) and put in *Bad Mom's 2*. The movie was the only reason I made it 45 min on the elliptical. I went and saw it in the theaters with my friends, and I remember it being funny, but forgot how funny it was. If you don't own both movies, you really need too.

I was active for 145 min and got in 12,062 steps.

<u>*Medicine and Vitamins*</u>

All meds on time... (I was even up to take my morning meds, and then went back to sleeping).

<u>*Energy and Symptoms*</u>

I got in 8 hours of shitty sleep. I didn't even have a good chunk of time. It is always a hit or miss with the doxepin. I hate that it leaves me so groggy the next day too. It's almost not even worth taking unless I have gone several nights with little too no sleep. I also spent most of the night flipping from side to side instead of sleeping on my back. My son came in at about 5am, and he was moving so much and that didn't help either.

When I finally dragged my ass out of bed, I went right for the spark. I knew that I would need that pick me up. I had some breakfast, but only 1 piece toast because if I ate 2, I would have been full and crawled back into bed for more sleep. I needed to move my body as well, so I started to meal prep my breakfast for the week. And since all my containers were still being used, I had the hubby run to Costco for some more.

After that was all said and done, I had another spark because I was still dragging ass. I cleaned up the kitchen and got laundry going. I noticed in the bathroom we had those stupid fucking winter ants (I don't know what they are called, but to me they are winter ants) everywhere. I HATE THEM SO MUCH. I noticed some ants in my writing area, but it was only 1 ant every day, for the past week and a half. I should have gotten the ant traps sooner. Made a trip to home depot and those little pests should be out of here in no time.

Today was very uneventful. I took it as a semi-rest day (because I still had shit to do, I was just in no hurry to get it done and I left some of the things that needed to get done for tomorrow).

I had no back pain and no fibro pain today. I was super exhausted, but that was from the doxepin. Tomorrow should be a great day. I will be all rested up and ready to go for the week. I am looking forward to getting some jogging in and picking up my workouts.

Day 28: March 5, 2018

Food Consumed

<u>Breakfast:</u> Hash browns with onions and 1 piece of homemade toast

<u>Snack:</u> Black bean chips

<u>Lunch:</u> Edamame and 4 tacos (rice and beans, vegan sour cream, avocado, lime juice and sriracha)

<u>Snack:</u> Multigrain tortilla chips

<u>Dinner:</u> Penne noodles with a little bit of olive oil and garlic salt and garlic bread

<u>Snack:</u> 3 chocolate chip cookies (I need to make more of these tomorrow. nom nom nom).

<u>Beverages:</u> Water= 86 fl. oz. Spark= 10 fl. oz.

Activity Level

We got ready for the day and I decided since it was P.E. day for my little guy, we would go to the track and do a workout together. It was nice out but still cold, so we bundled up and headed to the track after he finished up a few subjects in school. I walked 1 lap: jogged 100m, walked 100m (1 lap): jogged 200m, walked 200m: jogged 400m, walked 400m: jogged for 10 min (.95 miles).

I should have worn my leg warmers, they seem to make the cold more bearable. But did a good workout. I was nervous about jogging for 10 min. And by jogging, I mean I look like I am running behind a toddler. So, most people can run a mile in 10 min (.95 miles, but really close, so I'm gonna call it a mile). My previous mile times (even with the back pain) were between 7-8 min. I am going to take this as a win, because I know I have a long way to go and running that fast is going to take some time and training. I am happy to say that my back didn't hurt nor did any other part of my body. I finally feel like I can start running and I will be able to do a 10k this summer (or maybe even a half marathon). There was some slight discomfort with running, but I kept engaging my core and letting it go, so my brain could recognize that running will not hurt me. I will stay with the track workout and not run for more than 10 min this week. And if all goes well, I will bring that running time up to 15 min and hopefully throw in some very light weight training with it. I still have problems lifting heavy things, so I will not be pushing to hard for that.

I was active for 96 min and got in 10,363 steps. (I just want to point out that I am KILLING it on my steps the last few days.)

Medicine and Vitamins

All the meds. All on time. All about keeping it consistent.

<u>*Energy and Symptoms*</u>

I had a hard time falling asleep last night. My mind was racing like crazy. I was hoping that reading would help, but my mind kept distracting me from that and then I couldn't remember what I read. So, I put the book down and just tried to go to sleep, repeating affirmations in my head. It must have taken me about 40 min to finally fall asleep. After that, I slept pretty good. I was able to get in 7 hours of good sleep.

I woke up and thought I would have sometime to myself, but my littlest was already up and in the living room watching TV. I did sleep in until 8am, so I guess I lost this time.

I had great energy today and I had no pain. I feel like I should explain this "no pain" feeling that I have. I can't say that I have "no pain" when in honesty there is always a hinge or two here and there. From the pain I used to have that was almost debilitating to having an average pain of 5 daily, to now saying I have no pain. I mean that the pain I have in the "no pain" moments would be a level 2 pain to a person who never experiences pain on a daily basis. It does not prohibit me from going about my day and it doesn't slow me down at all. It is sometimes there, but I often forget about it unless I make a wrong move or try to pick up something heavy. So, this to me is "no pain." The only fibro pain that I have been feeling is when my arms start to get really cold when I am sitting in bed at night reading, but it goes away when I put on a sweater (I told you my body does not do good when it is cold).

I have 21 days left on this journey and I am excited for what those days hold in store for me.

Day 29: March 6, 2018

Food Consumed

Breakfast: 2 pieces of homemade toast

Snack: Multigrain tortilla chips

Lunch: Brown rice and quinoa with brussels sprouts and carrots

Snack: none (running around doing errands)

Dinner: Hash browns and 2 pieces of homemade toast

Snack: Coconut butter pecan ice cream

Beverages: Water= 72 fl. oz. Spark= 10 fl. oz.

Activity Level

It was so nice out today, so I walked from my therapist's office to meet my husband a couple miles away. It was warm enough too, that it wasn't making my muscles tense. I walked for 15 min and then decided to try jogging. I didn't want to jog on the pavement, I wanted to take this week and do it on the track but wasn't going to be able to make it to the track today, so I did what I had to do. So far, I am doing great. I only jogged for 11 min, so it wasn't too bad. I have some minor pain, but not enough to stop me from doing anything. Just having to be careful when I am bending over and stuff.

I was active for 103 min and got in 10,248 steps.

Medicine and Vitamins

Again…On time with all. Look at me killing it at adulting. I know that I have to be on these meds for the rest of my life, but maybe they will "perfect" adrenal transplants soon and I won't have to be on meds any more.

Appointments

Finally!! My bitch it out session with my amazing therapist. I haven't gone in 2 weeks and that was too long. I needed a bitch it out session to get a lot off my chest and the things that I am holding back on because I put everyone else who shouldn't be first, first. Lots of stress reduced and I got to take a walk in the sun.

Energy and Symptoms

Got in a big ol' chunk of sleep last night, and then little bit of shitty sleep, and then another good chunk. I woke up at 8am again. My son was up and watching TV in the living room. I think our roles have shifted and I need it to shift back. I can only blame myself this morning, because I did wake up at 6am and I was still a little tired and forced myself to go back to sleep. I could have gotten up and enjoyed some quiet time, so that is my fault for choosing to stay in my nice cozy bed.

I needed a bit of a change, since apparently coloring my hair wasn't enough, so I went and got it trimmed, but had her go a bit shorter this time. My hair grew so fast (another benefit from doing WFPB) in just 6 weeks. It grew a little over an inch. For some people, that might be nothing, but for me it usually takes my hair about 6 months to grow an inch. I will be going grey and letting it grow out. My oldest graduates in June and I want to see how long it will be at that time.

I feel like I did so many errands today that I didn't have time to get my stuff done, and then I started stressing about it. Trying to not stress about it and just chalking it up to a day that I can push things back. I was able to let go of what I couldn't control. Then my son had his big game today (playing at the college so recruiters could come see him), and then I was stressing about not being able to make it down to see him and now he is playing, and I am nervous for him. My face is feeling a little numb and my chest keeps getting heavy, as I am being updated on his playing stats. I am so proud of him. Mom stuff gets me more stressed than anything else, and that shit you can't just push to the side and let go. So, I am ok with that stress, but my body isn't.

Another good day down and a life time more to go. Still learning things and growing. I will be trying some new recipes (I am sure you are tired of seeing the same things I eat over and over, but I am not tired of eating them). If I can get my "stresses" under control, I think it will make things a lot easier as well.

Day 30: March 7, 2018

Food Consumed

Breakfast: 2 pieces of homemade toast with peanut butter

Snack: Avocado and multigrain tortilla chips

Lunch: Edamame

Snack: none

Dinner: Brown rice and quinoa with shrimp (had to get rid of it so don't be all judgy).

Snack: 2 homemade chocolate chip cookies

Beverages: Water= 84 fl. oz. Spark= 10 fl. oz.

Activity Level

I was active for 50 min and got in 4,164 steps (My day was shit).

Medicine and Vitamins

I did get all my meds on time, so I guess I am winning at that.

Appointments

My youngest son went in for his allergy shots and I got the results back from my blood draw back in February. The results from my blood test weren't great. It was when I had my crisis and my levels were horrible. My DHEA levels were crazy low, my Ferritin (iron storage) levels were really high which means infection or inflammation, my liver was being sluggish, and my kidneys were trying to keep up with being dehydrated (even though I was drinking plenty of water, my body just wasn't absorbing it). It was a good thing I went in, that I knew I needed to stress dose, and I made sure I was resting. This could have been a lot worse if I had just tried to ignore it (like I have done in the past). It is really scary to see your levels that low and knowing that your body can shut down so fast and easily. I can't stress how important it is to make sure that when you feel the slightest difference in what your body is doing to stress dose, talk to your endocrinologist and know what to do to prevent an adrenal crisis from becoming fatal.

Energy and Symptoms

I do not know what I ate yesterday (of course I do, it's right up there in yesterdays journaling- duh!), but it gave me gas all night and all day today. It was awful, but there is nothing to do but let it out.

I didn't sleep well, only got in 5 ½ hours. I don't know what was going on, but I just kept waking up and I was really uncomfortable. I think I am going to try to stay on my back with an extra pillow to prop me up a little. That left shoulder is still bothering me. I don't know why it has become so painful, but I need to get that looked at.

Today, I think we all should have just stayed in bed. My littlest took 3 hours…. 3 HOURS!!! To do 2 pages in math. That was only 40 math problems that he can usually do in 15-30 min. But today he thought it would be more productive to stare at nothing, to play with the pencil, to recite god knows what in his head. Took away all his electronics, his Beyblades, and his bedtime TV time. Still didn't phase him. He didn't get done with his school work until 5:20pm. Let's just say that caused me some stress, that it had my face numb and twitching. I was having some heaviness in my chest and I was just trying to let him be. So instead of sitting next to him, I went and got my stuff done that needed to be done, but I was still so upset with him. It's almost worth putting him back in school and just letting him fail on his own and he can be in 3rd grade for 5 more years. Until he understands that he can't just choose to not do his work….. Vent over.

I didn't get in any workout today, I didn't reach my step or activity goal, but I did still get a lot of computer/author/wife/mom stuff done, so I guess I will take that as a win. I have no choice…Right?

I have been slacking on getting all the meal/snacks in, but still doing pretty good. Tonight, I was going through our freezer stuff and I still have some shrimp and fish in there that needs to be eaten before it goes bad, so I made some shrimp. I love shrimp so much, it has always been my favorite. After having it tonight, I can live without it. I don't miss it, I didn't LOVE it. It was just ok. I just hope it sits well with me. I would hate to get sick or have a flare from it. I know that I can now live without it. Sometimes you get that thought that you might miss certain meats and stuff. So far, I have had the shrimp and the sushi and I know that I can live without it and I won't miss it. Looking at meats though. It makes me a little sick to my stomach. I don't even like the smell of it any more.

Other than the stress my son caused me today, I think it was a pretty decent day. About a level 2 with back pain (I was doing a lot of bending over today), but nothing that was hindering me from doing anything. I only had a tiny bit of fibro pain and that was because I was cold and that was only like a level 2.

Day 31: March 8, 2018

Food Consumed

Breakfast: 2 pieces of homemade toast with peanut butter

Snack: none (speech therapy for my son)

Lunch: 4 tacos (corn tortilla, vegan sour cream, avocado, brown rice, quinoa, and beans, sriracha)

Snack: none (fighting with my son on school work)

Dinner: Hash browns and 2 pieces of homemade toast

Snack: 2 amazing homemade chocolate chip yumminess cookies

Beverages: Water= 80 fl. oz. Spark= 10 fl. oz.

Activity Level

I got on the elliptical and was lucky enough to get in 40 min. I wanted to do more with the workout, but since everything got pushed back today, I had to be a responsible mom and make dinner.

I was active for 86 min and got in 8,048 steps.

Medicine and Vitamins

With how the day went, I was still able to focus enough to get my meds taken on time.

Energy and Symptoms

I was hurting pretty bad last night. My fault for eating the shrimp, but it was just not a fun night to try and sleep. My body was not happy, and my mind was racing like crazy. I did not wear my ear plugs last night and my youngest was in my bed by the time I crawled into it. He got up 3 times last night before he finally went back to his own bed. I got 6 hours but felt like I only got 2. I was fine once I was up and moving, but if it hadn't been for my son waking me up and making me get out of bed, I would have stayed there all day.

Got up and moving and then I was fine. I had great energy and got ready to take my son to speech therapy. Not before having another amazing morning of math with him. 2 days in a row of "fuck you. I'm not wanting to do math." He started at 8:40am, worked on math until we had to leave for speech at 10:30am. Got home and he started working on math again at 12:45pm and didn't finish until 3pm. Talk about stressing the fuck out. I even tried to ignore it today, but I am not good at that and it really gets to me. More face numbness and twitching and I could feel my body starting to ache. I might have to start stress dosing just to get him through school if something doesn't change (trying something new next week to help-the both of us).

With him taking so long with that, I wasn't able to get everything I wanted done, but did get most of it, so that's good. I started to stress about newsletters and websites, on top of this difficult child, and not being able to get to the track for a workout, because it was a monsoon outside. It was just not my day. I didn't eat like I was supposed too, so I missed out on 2 snack times.

After my shower tonight, exhaustion hit hard. I am so ready to crawl in bed and it's only 7pm. I still have a lot of mom shit left to do. My back pain today was about a level 3.

I heard from one of my friends who is doing the WFPB plan. She is doing ok on it. She has had a couple bad days and she has only been doing it for 10 days. She did notice that she didn't feel like she needed a nap for the past couple days. Pain has been the same. She is going to adjust her bread intake. She thinks that she has had more consistent pain with having the added bread to her diet. She is going to take bread out for a couple days and then try gluten free bread and see how that works for her. She is enjoying the food and her skin is feeling amazing.

Today is day 30 for my son just doing the no dairy. I reminded him of his results and how he has been feeling and that I really hope he sticks with it. He told me that he might go off of it to see what happens and if it's bad then he will go back to being dairy free. I can't wait to hear how his first time with dairy goes after not having it for a while. I told him he is going to feel like shit and have the fast potties (aka diarrhea). So hard to make teenagers step away from their sacred pizza.

My other friend who is doing the WFPB is struggling with giving up cheese. She can't seem to let it go and it is what is making her feel like shit. She eats it and feels awful but can't give it up. She is going through other life stresses and I think at this time trying to fit this plan into all of that chaos is just too much right now. And that is ok, sometimes you need to get your shit together in order to start something new and there is nothing wrong with that.

I am so looking forward to this day being over and starting new tomorrow.

Day 32: March 09, 2018

Food Consumed

Breakfast: 2 pieces of homemade toast with peanut butter

Snack: None (PT/chiro)

Lunch: Edamame

Snack: Pistachios, applesauce, carrots, and multigrain tortilla chips

Dinner: 2 pieces of homemade pizza (vegan cheese with vegan ranch dressing)

Snack: None (basketball game and working on marketing)

Beverages: Water= 80 fl. oz. Spark= 10 fl. oz.

Activity Level

Put on a movie and did 60 min on the Elliptical. I was active for 115 min and got in 9,866 steps.

Medicine and Vitamins

I took my all my meds on time today (signing and a happy dance).

Appointments

I had my PT/Chiro appointment early this morning. It was so nice to have soft tissue work done. I wish that was the whole appointment. With the stress my body has been through the past couple days (not to mention shitty sleep), I need some good soft tissue work done.

Energy and Symptoms

I didn't sleep all that great last night, but it was better than the night before. I remembered to put in my ear plugs. I had a rough time falling asleep and I had propped myself up, which didn't work like I wanted it to. My upper back was killing me this morning. I was up at 8am though, semi ready to take on the day.

I was so happy that we did not have to go through the whole "school" thing today. I don't think I could have made it through another rough day.

After my PT/Chiro appointment, I decided I needed to do some major prep for my book stuff and finally set up my website and all the things authors need to do. I sent my youngest to play on the computer and I got shit done. It feels good (as I sit her at 1am) to have it done, up, and going. It was frustrating and overwhelming, but I knew it needed to be done. My shoulders, neck, and back are killing me from being at the computer all day. I did take an hour break to workout. I didn't want to miss out on that opportunity. Do I feel bad that I had my son playing video games all day?...... Not one bit.

Again, I didn't eat very well. Having to get everything done in one day is not fun, and eating was what I put on the back burner. My brain feels like mush and I am sure I forgot to do at least 5 things, but that can all be done tomorrow. My body has had enough today.

I did get a break from being in front of the computer for a while. We ended up going to a friend's son's basketball game. My ass did not like the bleachers tonight. My low back started to hurt more and when we were leaving I stepped off the steep sidewalk and it jolted my back. That fucking hurt and I had a hard time getting in the car. I iced when I got home, but it is bothering me. My body pain level today is a 6 and climbing right now. My shoulders feel like they are on fire, my joints are all hurting, and my muscles feel like they ran a marathon. Today is not a good day and I know it is my fault sitting for a good portion of the day. My body cannot handle this, but I had to get things done. I will sleep it off tonight and not be so harsh on it tomorrow.

Day 33: March 10, 2018

Food Consumed

Breakfast: 2 pieces of homemade toast with peanut butter

Snack: none (slept until 10am-late breakfast)

Lunch: Edamame and applesauce

Snack: Pistachios and multigrain tortilla chips

Dinner: Hash browns and 2 pieces of homemade toast

Snack: 2 homemade chocolate chip cookies

Beverages: Water= 104 fl. oz. Spark= 10 fl. oz.

Activity Level

I got up and the sun was begging me to come out and play. I ate a little breakfast and then headed to the track. I walked a lap, ran for 15 min, and then walked for 28 min. It felt so good, but I was tired. I was surprised I made it 1.55 miles. My back didn't hurt while I was jogging, and I didn't have to really engage my core. With how bad my body was last night, I was really surprised it held up during the run. Did about 100m of lunges and walked the rest of the time. Stretched out really good when I got home.

I was active for 159 min and got in 16,277 steps.

Medicine and Vitamins

On time today. I also had to stress dose (gonna party hard tonight, so I need to be prepared).

Energy and Symptoms

I was up past 2am. Laid in bed forever trying to fall asleep. It just didn't come easy. I was in a lot of pain. I do not know what caused the flare, but my body was so pissed. I got about 4 hours total of sleep. I was up at 6am and could not fall back asleep until about 8:30am. It was rough.

when I got home from the track, I jumped back on the computer to finish up with stuff that was left from last night.

Being in front of the computer for 2 days has really taken a toll on my body and eyes. I have the worst headache and ended up having to take 800mg of ibuprofen. I am going out with the girls tonight for my friends Dirty 30. We are going to a dance club at a casino, so I needed to stress dose for that. Since I can't drink, I won't be dancing as much, but still taking precaution with how my body will handle what I will be doing.

I haven't been out like this since I went to Vegas in October and I didn't even dance then. There was just A LOT of walking. I am excited to go out but nervous as well. I do not do well in crowds, people annoy the shit out of me, and being in a closed area with smokers is going to be really hard. My body just doesn't handle things as well as it used too, but it will be fun to let loose with my ladies.

Day 34: March 11, 2018

Food Consumed

Breakfast: 1-piece homemade toast with peanut butter

Snack: none (slept in and had breakfast at 11am)

Lunch: Edamame

Snack: Carrots and multigrain tortilla chips

Dinner: 5 tacos (brown rice and quinoa and beans, avocado, vegan sour cream and corn tortillas and sriracha)

Snack: 2 homemade chocolate chip cookies

Beverages: Water= 80 fl. oz. Spark= 10 fl. oz.

Activity Level

Even with being exhausted, I went out and mowed the front yard (thank you spark). I was a little nervous since every time I did it last year, I would be in pain for a few hours after. This time I was fine during and after. It only took me 20 min to get the front yard done. It was so nice the last couple days and our grass was looking so gross, I wanted to get out before it started to rain again (this is Western Washington, so the odds of rain are VERY high).

I was active for 134 min and got in 11,158 steps

<u>*Medicine and Vitamins*</u>

I was late taking my morning meds because I slept in, but on time the rest of the day. Just couldn't get moving this morning.

<u>*Energy and Symptoms*</u>

I didn't sleep very well, but I did sleep in until about 10:20am. Which means I missed my morning med time (and I was on a roll). My tracker said I got about 4 ½ hours of sleep. It sure feels like that too. Woke up with PGV (party girl voice), but there was no PG-ing. No drinking for me (besides the 2 water bottles I downed). My throat was hurting pretty bad all day (I think it was from all the cigarette smoke). I hate that they allow smoking in the club.

After mowing, I showered, got dressed, and took a very short "nap" (laid there for about 30 min trying to fall asleep). I have felt like a zombie all day. I can't complain too much because I have not had pain today, just the exhaustion. The girls came over and then we headed for the Casino for a night of dancing. It was a lot of fun. My body held up through the dancing. I was sweating so bad, I was soaked. My hair was so wet it kept dripping on me. I had to wipe myself down with a few napkins. I am so glad I ended up wearing a tank top instead of the ¾ sleeve sweater that I had on. My tank top was drenched. That just means I had a lot of fun. I got home about 2am and I was exhausted.

The WFPB plan is working, but I know that I still can't go out until 2am on a shitty nights sleep, sleep shitty again, and then try to function (during daylight savings). I don't think even a healthy person could do that, but I had a lot of fun and I am looking forward to more nights like this (just maybe not being out until 2am).

Day 35: March 12, 2018

Food Consumed

Breakfast: 1 piece of homemade toast with peanut butter

Snack: None (had a late breakfast)

Lunch: Carrots, edamame, and applesauce

Snack: Multigrain tortilla chips with an avocado

Dinner: Hash browns and 2 pieces of homemade toast

Snack: None (busy on website and forgot)

Beverages: Water= 80 fl. oz. Spark= 10 fl. oz.

Activity Level

We went for a walk around the track for PE, and my son got to ride his scooter. It was such a beautiful day out, we had to get out and enjoy it. I jogged for 15 min and it felt really good. I wish I could have ran longer, but I have to take it slow.

We ended up taking the dogs for a walk as well. The dogs were super excited. We have leashes that we use so the dogs don't walk us, but they hate them. It is nice that I don't have to fight against a 90lb dog who is pulling. So much better on my body and my son can easily walk our 50lb dog without her pulling him.

I was active for 80 mins and got in 9,007 steps.

<u>*Medicine and Vitamins*</u>

Meds were all taken on time today. YAY!!

<u>*Energy and Symptoms*</u>

I thought I slept good last night, but I guess I didn't. Had a hard time falling asleep. Restarted my audio book 3 times for 30 min intervals. I slept on my back and ended up moving to my side because of the pain in my shoulder. I did put a pillow under my side to help align my back better and that seemed to work great, but I must have tossed back and forth a lot (according to my sleep tracker). My youngest was also in bed with me, so that might have played a big role in how I slept. I didn't have my ear plugs in either.

We got up around 8:20am, but we were still tired, so we went back to bed and laid there until 9:30am. I don't mind having mornings like that. When my little guy needs more rest, and I was still feeling exhausted, it's ok to just crawl back into a nice warm bed and cuddle.

He did a lot better with school today and we got done at the normal 3pm time. No stress for this mama today.

Lots of vitamin D and it really helps with the mood. I noticed that both times I was out, that my allergies were kicking in. I haven't had any issues with allergies for 3 years. I need to get back in and get some allergy shots. Something must have changed this year, which is not good for me. My throat is still bothering me a bit (I think the cigarette smoke is still hanging on).

Today was a great day. I had no pain, no fibro pain, I ran for 15 min and felt great after. Part of the run was on the pavement too. Didn't have stress today with my son's school, got all my goals met, the house didn't need much attention, I got some sun. It was a great day. Hopefully sleep will be just as good.

Day 36: March 13, 2018

Food Consumed

Breakfast: 1 ½ pieces of homemade toast with peanut butter

Snack: none (my throat was hurting so bad, it hurt to eat)

Lunch: Avocado and multigrain tortilla chips (very little, throat was still pretty sore)

Snack: Apple sauce

Dinner: Rice and mixed veggies

Snack: 2 homemade chocolate chip cookies

Beverages: Water= 80 fl. oz. Spark= 20 fl. oz.

Activity Level

After therapy I jogged home. I was only planning on jogging for 15 min, but my body was feeling some stress and it didn't want to stop running, it was begging to get the stress out, so I let it go for as long as it wanted to (which happened to be all the way home- 4.8 miles in 50 min). I didn't fatigue, I didn't struggle, it just felt amazing to run. I was worried that I might start hurting once I stopped, but my back never started to hurt.

I was active for 111 min and got in 13,173 steps.

<u>*Medicine and Vitamins*</u>

I was late for my afternoon meds because I was running. It was only by 30 min so that wasn't to bad. I ended up stress dosing for my last two doses.

<u>*Appointments*</u>

Great session with therapy; always brings me back to a manageable stress level. It's my favorite day of the week. I get out all my frustrations and she brings me back to a "reset" for the rest of the week.

<u>*Energy and Symptoms*</u>

My sleep has been taking a hit and I can't figure out why. This is sucks so bad. I got 5 hours and 20 min last night. I tossed and turned and just couldn't get into a deep enough sleep. I really wanted to just stay in bed. My throat was hurting really bad and I was just so exhausted.

Started to get my youngest going for school and getting myself ready to go to therapy. My ex called and there was some drama going on. I was trying to not let it affect me and just trying to keep the peace. When we are told 2 different things, it really puts us both on edge and it's something that my body does not need when it's already fighting against itself. Hopefully we can just keep things good and communicate better.

The only thing that was awful and had me down was my allergies. My eyes were so red, it was scary looking. I was sneezing like crazy (no back pain with the sneezing. YAY!!) and itchy watery eyes. I called my naturopath to see if I could come get allergy shots (haven't had any issues in 2-3 years), and they are out of the actual allergen stuff and had to order more…. It won't be here for 4-5 weeks (crying internally). Not sure my body can take it. I believe since it is fighting the allergies and the sore throat, it's weak right now and that is why I am so exhausted. The diet change could be the reason for the allergies too. Sometimes the change in eating habits can bring about a change in the immune system and not always for the better. Not that allergies are as bad as an autoimmune disease, but they are not fun.

I ate shitty today again. My throat was just not happy, so I didn't need to be pissing it off anymore than it was. I really need to sleep good so I can heal. Is there a pill out there that can put me in a coma?? Where can I get it??

I wouldn't say I am having a "flare", but I am definitely feeling a bit run down and slight achiness in my body. Like I said above, right now it is fighting something, so it is needing rest.

Day 37: March 14, 2018

Food Consumed

Breakfast: Hash browns and 1 piece of homemade toast

Snack: none (late breakfast because I had PT/Chiro so early)

Lunch: Edamame

Snack: Multigrain tortilla chips and pistachios

Dinner: 5 tacos (brown rice, quinoa, and beans, vegan sour cream, avocados, and sriracha)

Snack: 2 homemade chocolate chip cookies

Beverages: Water= 80 fl. oz.

Activity Level

Was at PT (their office) for 38 min. I went for a walk with the dogs for 22 min. That is a great arm workout. Even though the leashes they have don't allow them to pull, they still pull enough to give the arms a little workout.

I was active for 126 min and got in 8,153 steps.

Medicine and Vitamins

I got all my meds in my body on time.

Appointments

PT and Chiro. It felt good to get in some exercise and release a little on my back. Always feels good to get adjusted. I wish I could do that every other day.

Energy and Symptoms

I slept ok last night. I got in 6 ½ hours, but it was really interrupted. I managed to arrange all the pillows so that my lower back didn't hurt, which was nice. I had to be up early for my PT/Chiro appointment (I hate early appointments). I really just wanted to sleep in, but I was glad that I got the day going with some exercise. Even better, I woke up with no pain from my run yesterday, not even soreness. This means that I CAN RUN!!!! I am so excited.

Today was a stress-free day and was really nice. My youngest started Special Olympics swim. He did amazing at his first practice. It was really fun to watch him do something that he loves so much. He worked really hard to get done with his school work, which was really nice. He was focused and very happy.

Today went by so fast. The weather cleared up, so we decided to take our dogs for a walk. My allergies are still really bad and I can't wait for the shots so this hell can be over with. It is what is causing my exhaustion. My throat does feel better today though, so that is a plus.

I had just minor annoying pain in my back while I was walking the dogs, but other than that it was really good day. No fibro pain at all, just exhaustion from my body fighting allergies and that is from the Addison's.

Day 38: March 15, 2018

Food Consumed

<u>Breakfast:</u> 2 pieces of homemade toast with peanut butter

<u>Snack:</u> Apple sauce

<u>Lunch:</u> Edamame and multigrain tortilla chips

<u>Snack:</u> Pistachios

<u>Dinner:</u> Brown rice and quinoa with broccoli and zucchini

<u>Snack:</u> 2 chocolate chip cookies

<u>Beverages:</u> Water= 80 fl. oz. Spark= 10 fl. oz.

Activity Level

I was so glad that the weather was amazing. When I took my son to speech therapy, I decided to go for a run (I ran 4 miles in 39 min). It felt so amazing. I also signed up for 2 races (one in April and one in May). I am only doing the 10k instead of the half marathon, but I think I might change the one in May to a half. This is very exciting for me since it has been so long since I have been able to run without pain. I think I actually had a smile on my face the whole time (probably looked crazy to everyone who drove past me). My older 2 sons' will be doing the April race too. I did the race 2 years ago and they came out to watch, but this year they will actually get to run it with me.

I was active for 107 min and got in 12,216

Medicine and Vitamins

All meds were taken on time. I took allergy meds and ibuprofen to help give my body a fighting chance against the pollen.

Energy and Symptoms

I did not sleep the best last night. I woke up pretty tired and didn't want to get out of bed. My youngest was in the bed with me and he slept until 9:30am. He must have needed it. I was up at 8:20am. I am so glad that I will be able to sleep in as long as I want tomorrow. I don't have anywhere to be until 1:30pm. I still have shit to do, but my body doesn't have to get up and do anything until it wants too, and I am going to take advantage of that.

Worked on book stuff today and of course vegged out to March Madness. I am doing amazing on my bracket and I am loving all the games. It is going to consume my life until April, but that's ok. I can always sit there with my laptop and let it distract me.

I had no stress today. It was nice. I had no pain and just the right amount of energy. I am going to need to charge up for tomorrow, because I do need to juice, make homemade bread and pasta sauce, and other meal prep stuff. I got this!

Day 39: March 16, 2018

Food Consumed

<u>Breakfast:</u> Grapenuts with rice milk (changed it up)

<u>Snack:</u> none (ate breakfast late)

<u>Lunch:</u> Edamame

<u>Snack:</u> Apple and almond butter

<u>Dinner:</u> Best fucking mac and cheese I have ever put in my mouth!!! HOMEMADE (WFPB recipe)

<u>Snack:</u> 2 chocolate chip cookies

<u>Beverages:</u> Water= 80 fl. oz. Spark= 10 fl. oz.

Activity Level

This sure took a hit today. I was active for 46 min and got in 3,379 steps

Medicine and Vitamins

All meds were taken on time, but it didn't help with giving me any kind of energy.

I didn't sleep well. I almost got 5 hours of horribly interrupted sleep. Lots of tossing and turning and waking up, it was a mess. Little guy was up early after not going to bed until after 2am. I was looking forward to sleeping in, but that didn't happen. I wanted to go back to bed at 10am, but that wasn't an option either. I made the most of what my body was producing, which was barely enough to hold my eyes open.

Got my spark in me and that didn't help much. I was able to get all the things I needed to for my book done while my little guy was at swim practice. I was planning on going for a run, but the allergies kicked in full force causing a horrible headache and extreme fatigue. I thought it would be best to stay inside and not suffer more than I had to with an already struggling body.

I did make 2 loaves of homemade bread (again…In the bread machines), homemade pasta sauce, and 1 pizza dough (ran out of flour), and I made homemade mac and cheese. Ok, so I have to talk about this WFPB recipe. I was really scared to make it. My youngest LOVES mac and cheese but is SUPER picky about it (he likes the boxed crap). So, we haven't had mac and cheese for a long time (I think it's been over a year). I wasn't sure how it would turn out and as I was making it, I was doubting it every step of the way. It didn't smell to appealing, but OMFG!!! It was the best thing EVER. My son LOVED it and said we should sell it to people (he's always trying to get me to sell all the foods I make that he loves). I was really happy about this recipe and it will be used at least twice a month.

I really wish I could have gotten in a workout of some sort today, but I really didn't want to push my body and I had zero motivation. That's not all true, I had motivation, I just didn't want to be scratching my eyes and sneezing like crazy. I could have done an in-home workout, but that is what I had no motivation for. Unless that exercise involved me, alone in bed, power napping.

Talked to my oldest son tonight and he told me he ended up having broccoli cheese soup, with some cheesy garlic bread and milk. I asked him how he felt after and he said, "not good." He was stopped up, bad stomach pains, he noticed the next day that his face had more breakouts to it and his allergies had came back. He was AMAZED that it all came back in just 1 day of having dairy. I am happy to say, that he is cutting out dairy as much as he possibly can. He likes how he felt off of it, but he will wean himself off milk and also not have it as much as he has. He also has been asked by several people, how do I get my protein if my diet is plant based. This made a great discussion for us about protein, and why animal protein is not good for us, and how all these different plants and nuts have all the good protein we need. I also sent him a couple pictures and lists of all the protein I am getting and from what plants and how much they contain per serving. Great discussion for him to have with others so that they might look into changing some of their habits and really taking a look at what they are putting in their bodies.

My body had no pain today. Just really exhausted. It was fine until the allergies kicked in and it had to fight against that attack. As good as this diet is, Addison's disease and its exhaustion, when my body is fighting, will always win. When I don't have to battle against allergies (or a cold- knock on wood), this diet is PERFECT. I am not complaining at all. I have suffered

enough and know that I would be 100x worse off had I not started the

WFPB plan.

Day 40: March 17, 2018

Food Consumed

Breakfast: none (slept until 11am)

Snack: none

Lunch: Left over homemade mac and cheese (didn't eat lunch until 2pm- kept forgetting to eat)

Snack: Banana

Dinner: Stir Fry (broccoli, carrots, red onion, green onion, mushrooms, zucchini, and garlic- white rice)

Snack: none

Beverages: Water= 80 fl. oz. Spark= 10 fl. oz.

Activity Level

Ran 4.57 miles around the track (43 min). I really didn't want to, but I forced myself to go and was very happy that I did. Running always makes things better.

I was active for 109 min and got in 12,826 steps

Medicine and Vitamins

I was late for all my meds except for the night one (add in some allergy meds too). That's what happens when you sleep until 11am. I guess my body really needed it, or maybe it was because I took Doxepin (Ya. It was the doxepin).

Energy and Symptoms

I think I slept ok. I took doxepin last night to aid me, but my tracker said it was off my wrist for 3 hours (which it wasn't), but I am pretty sure I slept that whole time. I did not want to get out of bed, but forced myself too (after 11am). That is why I hate taking the doxepin, but desperate times call for desperate measures.

When I got home from my run, I started getting all the meal prep stuff done that needed to be done. I knew if I sat down, I would fall asleep. And that is what happened when I got done. Around 3pm I sat (laid) down on the coach and fell asleep for about 20 min (but laid there for an hour). My youngest came and covered me up and then filled up my water bottle, so that when I woke up I could have water (this baby boy LOVES taking care of his mama). Got up because the timer went off for the stuff I had been cooking, and then I finished out the rest of meal prep and started dinner.

I ended up having to take some allergy meds today, and I think that helped aid in my grogginess. I am so ready for bed right now, but I have to jump in the shower. I have put if off since 1pm. It should be nice to go right from there to bed.

I didn't have any pain today and with meal prepping, it didn't affect my back like it had done the last few times. I am really happy about that. This exhaustion is killing me right now though. I am so ready to just call it a night, but adulting must be done first.

Day 41: March 18, 2018

Food Consumed

<u>Breakfast:</u> Bowl of grape nuts

<u>Snack:</u> 1 piece of peanut butter toast

<u>Lunch:</u> 5 tacos (vegan sour cream, guacamole, rice and beans, sriracha)

<u>Snack:</u> Mean green

<u>Dinner:</u> Pasta with homemade pasta sauce 1 piece of homemade garlic bread

<u>Snack:</u> 2 chocolate chip cookies

<u>Beverages:</u> Water= 88 fl. oz. Spark= 10 fl. oz. Mean green= 12 fl. oz.

Activity Level

I was so exhausted but wanted to get in a good run today (ran 5.64 miles in 54 min. 8 sec) and I needed to go get new running shoes. Went and got new running shoes (didn't realize how badly worn and pronated my shoes were until I put on the new ones. HUGE difference). My knee had been bothering me on my recent runs, and with the new shoes (and the pronation correction), my knee didn't hurt, and I felt great.

I was active for 158 min and got in 16,019 steps

Medicine and Vitamins

Got all my meds taken on time. Took some allergy medicine (again). Hopefully these weeks will go by quickly and I can get my shots before this season kills me.

Energy and Symptoms

I slept for 5 hours and 40 min, but the longest I slept was an hour (before I was up tossing all night). I think I might try turning off my bed warmer and heater. I might be getting to hot and it's disrupting my sleep. I will narrow this down and figure it out. We had to be up early for my son's swim practice. He only lasted an hour because he didn't sleep well and was tired, plus he got hungry (might have to bring snacks-I fed him before we left though).

Came home and turned on some NCAA madness. My bracket is still holding up pretty good. Showered (since I was to exhausted last night-I'm so gross), and then got to doing my Sunday cleaning. My body was starting to feel the effects from the run. The allergy meds are really exhausting me. They are supposed to be non-drowsy, but I can definitely tell they are making me sleepy.

I have been on my feet all day and about 7pm, my feet and legs said that it is. They started hurting and it has been very difficult to walk. I massaged them for a little bit (my poor hands couldn't do much), and I had them elevated, but I am sure feeling the pain. I have done pretty good all day, but it was just too much on me today.

During my run (about mile 3), I was starting to feel about a 3-level pain in my back, but it didn't get worse, so I kept going. My hips are in a bit of pain right now, but I stretched really good. I think my body is just not liking how much it was used today. I am in need of a really good nights sleep (for a few nights) and to have these allergies done. My body can't keep fighting hard like this, it is setting me back a bit. I am still up and going, still able to do life and adult, so that is really good.

Day 42: March 19, 2018

Food Consumed

Breakfast: Grape nuts

Snack: none (took a nap)

Lunch: Leftover stir fry

Snack: none (fighting a migraine)

Dinner: 5 tacos (vegan sour cream, avocado, rice and beans, and sriracha)

Snack: 2 homemade cookies

Beverages: Water= 100 fl. oz. Mean green= 10 fl. oz.

Activity Level

I was only active for 21 mins and got in 1,742 steps. It was a rough day.

Medicine and Vitamins

Got my morning meds on time, was an hour late for my afternoon dose, and the rest were on time.

Energy and Symptoms

Slept really shitty last night. Having the heater and bed warmer off, didn't change anything. I felt like I didn't even fall asleep, but my sleep tracker says I got in 6 ½ hours. Got up and started homeschooling, but my exhaustion kept getting worse. I ended up having to take a nap. I laid down from 11:45am-1:30pm. I rested, but not sure if I actually slept.

Got up and my head was pounding, my allergies were hitting me hard. I laid around all day. My vison was blurry because my head was so bad. I could barely get around.

There was no fibro pain, but the Addisons disease is kicking my ass along with the allergies. Hoping for a better day tomorrow. I know I over did it yesterday and I think this whole week, with battling the pollen, has just taken me out. I was not counting on how badly my body would react to having allergies again.

Day 43: March 20, 2018

Food Consumed

<u>Breakfast:</u> 2 homemade pieces of peanut butter toast

<u>Snack:</u> Banana

<u>Lunch:</u> Edamame

<u>Snack:</u> Apple and almond butter

<u>Dinner:</u> Cream of wheat

<u>Snack:</u> 1 homemade chocolate chip cookie

<u>Beverages:</u> Water= 80 fl. oz. Coconut water= 8 fl. oz. Mean green= 12 fl. oz.

Activity Level

Today, since yesterday was horrific, I only ran 3 miles. I didn't want to push my already weak body. It did really good on the run though. I felt great and I really wanted to run more, but I was good and just kept to my 3.02 miles (30:34 min and walked 1.17 miles in 17:53 min). Allergies were under control (for a few hours after the run anyways).

 I was active for 120 min and got in 12,861 steps.

Medicine and Vitamins

Meds. Check… All on time… Check! Look at me. I know it's not consistent, but I have to give myself some credit for getting them taken on time.

Appointments

I had therapy (I don't know what I would do if I wasn't able to go in and bitch it out every week).

Energy and Symptoms

Surprise, surprise. Another night of shitty sleep. I need to do the kiwi's again. Those seemed to help and that is the only thing that has changed since I was getting good sleep. I had to pretty much overdose on allergy meds and I also took 800mg of ibuprofen (DO NOT TRY THIS AT HOME). It got me through the day.

Had great energy the rest of the day. It wasn't too eventful. Got some things done around the house and did some book stuff and blogging. Looked at some recipes (I know you are all tired of seeing my diet the same…Every day). I am branching out (and always thinking of the mac and cheese I made the other night-go to my blog for the recipe-www.chronicmomsclub.wixsite.com/chronicmomsclub).

No pain from running today, still no fibro pain. I am doing great and feeling amazing (minus the stupid allergy stuff, but I don't want to talk about that). I could have easily given myself 30 days on this diet and had my mind changed, shit I could have given myself 10 days on this diet and had my mind changed (not diet-lifestyle). I am sad that my 50 days are almost up, and I won't be documenting it anymore for people to read. I will still be doing updates on my blog about it, because I think a year from now, I will have more recipes under my belt, I will be having 1-2 bad days a month (if that), and I will be running and working out and living the life that I have missed out on for almost 4 years now. It is really worth giving up shitty food.

Day 44: March 21, 2018

Food Consumed

Breakfast: Grape nuts

Snack: Pistachios and multigrain tortilla chips

Lunch: Edamame and apple sauce

Snack: none (swim practice)

Dinner: 6 tacos (vegan sour cream, cilantro, avocado, rice, lime juice, and sriracha)

Snack: 1 homemade chocolate chip cookie

Beverages: Water= 80 fl. oz. Spark= 10 fl. oz. Mean green= 10 fl. oz.

Activity Level

Got in my workout today. I only did 30 min on the elliptical and 10 min of PT moves (It was a very lazy workout). It was already 4pm and I was starting to feel exhausted. Having the sunroof open on the drive home from swim practice was enough to activate my allergies. Once they hit, exhaustion soon followed, but I pushed through and did a lazy workout, but at least it was a workout.

I was active for 96 min and got in 8,003 steps.

<u>*Medicine and Vitamins*</u>

All meds were taken on time!! Also had to take allergy meds. I hate taking them. They are not supposed to cause me to be sleepy and they do. Maybe I should try drowsy and see if that will give me some energy.

<u>*Energy and Symptoms*</u>

Between 12:36am-3:37am, I slept amazing. That's a plus. Wasn't able to fall back asleep until about 4:15am, because my husband was snoring…. Yes, I had in my ear plugs and could still hear him, and from there it was downhill. Lot's of tossing and turning. I did wake up feeling pretty refreshed though, so I guess it's not all bad.

I felt a little rushed today, but it was a nice easy day. My youngest had swim practice, so I was able to relax for that and just watch him.

The rest of the day I relaxed and watched a few of my shows. I have so many on DVR right now, it will take me MONTHS to catch up on everything. I can do that on the days my body needs rest.

Today I had minimal back pain, about a level 2. No fibro pain (YAY!!), and the exhaustion wasn't bad (because I wasn't outside enough-until the drive with the open sunroof). I was able to make it through my day and get the things I needed too, done. I just need to get this sleep thing figured out and get my allergy shots, then I should be great.

Day 45: March 22, 2018

Food Consumed

Breakfast: Cream of wheat

Snack: 1 piece of homemade peanut butter toast

Lunch: Edamame and chips

Snack: Pretzels

Dinner: 5 tacos (vegan sour cream, cilantro, avocado, rice, lime juice and sriracha)

Snack: 2 Homemade chocolate cookies

Beverages: Water= 80 fl. oz. Spark= 10 fl. oz. Mean green= 12 fl. oz. Cranberry juice= 16 fl. oz.

Activity Level

I went for a run today (ran 3 miles in 29:30 min), despite the fact that it was raining. I thought this would be a great "test" to see how my body would handle the cold weather on a run. I did wear my running mask and my beanie, layered up, and went out. I just went to the track that is close to my house, just in case I started to hurt bad and needed to get home quick. When I got to the track and did about 2 laps, the rain turned to tiny hail (the kind that stings when it hits you). I pulled up my running mask and kept going. LOVE that thing. I was able to run 3 miles and I did it just as fast as I have been running (even though I felt like I was going way slower). I didn't have any pain, I didn't feel stiff or sore, the fibro flare from cold weather didn't act up. I would say this was one of the best runs (as far as how my body felt) that I have done. Now I don't have to be afraid of running in the cold.

I was active for 92 min and got in 10,177 steps.

Medicine and Vitamins

All on time. Didn't have to take any allergy meds, because it was raining. I hate to say this, but I hope it keeps raining until I can get in for my shots.

Appointments

I went in for a massage today as well. It was eh. She wasn't great (my husband does a better job-since I have trained him to do so), but I guess I can't complain to much because she wasn't awful. I just wouldn't go back to her. It's so hard to find a good massage therapist who actually knows treatment and not just relaxation. I have had 3 massages in the past 3 months, and none have been worth going back too. I will go back to one of them for 2 reasons: 1- I have a membership and want to keep the price 2- She is from Dublin and has an amazing accent (she isn't a bad LMP, she just has a lot to learn about treatment, but does a good relaxation massage). I might try out a few Groupon places to see what is out there and hopefully find someone who is good.

It wasn't until about 3am that I finally got some good sleep and I slept until 7:20am. From about 11pm-3am was a little iffy. I am picking up some kiwi's tomorrow. I know they worked last time, so I am really hoping that they work this time. I did wake up feeling pretty refreshed though, so I guess that's not bad. Had a great flow of energy today. I wasn't high energy, but it was good, and I got shit done.

The rest of the day was just me stressing over the NCAA tournament. As long as my #1 pick keeps winning, I am good, but the team I had playing against them in the championship lost out today. Now, I just want the Zags to go all the way.

I am thankful that I am still doing great with keeping the fibro pain at bay. With it raining today, I didn't have any allergies to fight and I felt good. So, I know now that it is the stupid allergies that are kicking my Addison's into overdrive and making me so exhausted. Just a couple weeks left until I can get my shots and start getting them under control.

Day 46: March 23, 2018

Food Consumed

Breakfast: 1 piece of homemade toast with peanut butter

Snack: Mean green

Lunch: Tofu breakfast burrito (spinach tortilla, tofu, green onion, tomatoes, mushrooms, spinach, sriracha, and cilantro)

Snack: Pretzels from *Pretzel Time*

Dinner: Homemade pizza (sauce, artichokes, tomatoes, mushrooms, cilantro, spinach, and avocados)

Snack: 2 homemade chocolate chip cookies

Beverages: Water= 80 fl. oz. Mean green= 10 fl. oz.

Activity Level

We went through a 30 min PT workout and then he did some soft tissue work to try and get some blood flow going and muscles loosened up. He did WAY better job than the massage therapist.

I was active for 93 min and got in 5,186 steps.

Medicine and Vitamins

All on time. Yay me!

Appointments

Having early PT/chiro appointments is always hard. I don't mind working out in the mornings, but 9:30am is a little too early for me. Getting adjusted is fine, but the moving around doing exercise, is a bit much.

Energy and Symptoms

I got 5 hours and 45 min of sleep. It wasn't great. I didn't go to bed until after 12:30am. I had to get up at 8:45am which isn't bad, but I was up at 8am. I didn't feel like I was exhausted, so that was good. I did lay in bed until my alarm went off though.

I had every intention of working out today, but when I got home I got busy with stuff, like eating, and then had to take my son to swim, and then we had to go do errands, and then home to clean….Which didn't happen because I turned on the basketball games and watched them instead. I had a friend coming over to watch the Purdue game, so I didn't workout at all and nothing else got done. My friend complimented me on how amazing my skin looked. She said that it just looked healthier and like it was glowing. Which is funny, because I was looking at myself yesterday thinking I needed to get in for some microdermabrasion because my skin was looking pretty dull and gross.

I was excited that I did try two new recipes today. They turned out really good and they were quick and easy to make. Not that they would be enjoyed by my kids, but they can always be "modified" to be more "kid tasty."

Had movie night with my youngest, that didn't start until 10:30pm. I could tell he was fading about 11:15pm but he was fighting it. I was exhausted and just wanted to go to bed. I asked him if he was ready to just call it a night and go to bed… So, we went to bed. I wasn't about to fight him on getting him in his own bed, so I just let him sleep with me.

My back pain today was about a steady level 4 all day. I felt like I had to keep adjusting and it felt a little weak. I didn't have any fibro pain. It dropped about 20 degrees and snowed (I wasn't about to run in that). I think if it hadn't snowed I would have gone for a run. I did feel like I was cold all day though, so that could have contributed to the low back pain. I wasn't sure if eating a pretzel from *Pretzel Time* would cause me to have a flare or some reaction, but it didn't, so that was good. Still feeling pretty happy on this WFPB plan and that it is something easy and beneficial to continue to do.

Day 47: March 24, 2018

Food Consumed

Breakfast: Grape nuts

Snack: mean green

Lunch: 3 tacos (vegan sour cream, cilantro, rice, avocado, and sriracha) and edamame

Snack: Carrots and celery

Dinner: Vegan meatballs and chicken bites, carrots and cantaloupe.

Snack: 2 kiwis

Beverages: Water= 80 fl. oz. Spark= 10 fl. oz.

Activity Level

Didn't do shit today. Super lazy. Was active for 44 mins and got in 3,369.

Medicine and Vitamins

Slept in so I adjusted them all and took them an hour later than normal. I wouldn't call this on time, but then again, I would.

I slept pretty good last night. I did wake up and my allergies started bothering me, which then put me into exhaustion. I ended up taking a nap from 12:15pm until 1:30pm. I woke up and ate and then wanted to go right back down for a nap. Instead I tried to keep myself busy.

I gave myself a little facial and got ready to go to our friend's daughters B-day party. Nothing stresses me out more than having to buy a gift for a little girl. I have all boys, so I only have to buy a girl gift 1-2 times a year. I fucking hate it. They have so many choices and when you are given choices like "they like barbie dolls" "they like jewelry and stuff like that...." This doesn't help me. There are like 5,000 different "dolls" that can be considered barbie. Do they already have that doll? What kind of jewelry? All the "kid" jewelry looks so crappy, that I don't want to get them that kind of gift. It is WAY to stressful. I usually send my husband to do it, but he was working and I am always a last minute gift shopper for this kind of stuff.

I love hanging out with our friends and laughing. At these parties, our kids play, us adults talk and laugh, and it's relaxing.

I got home a cleaned, since I didn't have the energy to do it earlier, which was still exhausting. I finally got the kiwis yesterday, and I ate 2 tonight, so here's hoping for some sleep. My back felt a little stiff today, but not painful. Mid shoulders though, ugh! Those were not happy today. I just wish I would have had the energy to go for a run, because it was a beautiful day. Maybe some allergy meds and ibuprofen for tomorrow to help me out.

Day 48: March 25, 2018

Food Consumed

Breakfast: 1 piece of homemade bread with peanut butter

Snack: None (took an early nap instead)

Lunch: Edamame and hash browns

Snack: Pistachios and multigrain tortilla chips

Dinner: Pasta with homemade cashew fettucine sauce

Snack: 2 chocolate chip cookies and 2 kiwis

Beverages: Water= 120 fl. oz. Spark= 10 fl. oz.

Activity Level

When I got up, I got ready for a run. I wanted to do 6 miles. This was my goal. When I started, I didn't think I was going to make it 2 miles (all runners know that the first mile is a lie). I was going to call it good if I made it 4 miles. About mile 2, I said, I got this….6 miles is gonna be no problem. I did it. I hit my goal of 6 miles (62 min). I forgot though, when I was running, that on my way back home, it was going to be ALL UP HILL!!! That was exhausting and I feel that it killed my time a bit, but time wasn't my goal, the mileage was. I didn't hurt and it felt really good to put in that many miles. My goal for next month will be to run 7 miles.

I was active for 132 min and got in 16,083 steps.

<u>*Medicine and Vitamins*</u>

All meds on time. I feel like I am never going to be consistent with getting them in my body. I guess as long as they make it in me, I am good. Knowing that I was going on a long run today, I wanted to prepare myself, so I did take ibuprofen before I ran.

<u>*Energy and Symptoms*</u>

I got 5 hours and 20 min of sleep last night. VERY interrupted sleep, but I felt like I slept amazing. I was wide awake at 6:30am. Which is really weird, but I'll take it. I did go back to bed and slept from 8:30am-9:45am. I wasn't necessarily tired, I think it was more that I was just being lazy and wanted to be back in my warm bed.

I did some meal prep today and made more homemade bread. Nothing smells better than bread cooking. Tonight, for dinner I wanted to try out a new fettucine recipe. I had just enough cashews and nutritional yeast to make it. It didn't mix well (due to not going with my gut instinct of adding water slowly instead of all at once, so it was a little chunky). It was really good, and I actually liked the little chunks in it. My youngest had 3 bowls of it, so it was a hit. I hope it is as good warmed up the next day. I want it for lunch tomorrow, if my husband doesn't take it to work for his dinner.

The rest of the day I just cleaned house, watched the NCAA tournament, and was just kind of lazy. I didn't want to be on my feet all day after running 6 miles, so I listened to my body and took lots of long breaks, and just enjoying some college basketball.

I didn't have any fibro pain today and my low back pain was at a steady level 1. It was a really good day. Great food, great basketball, and very little pain. I call this a win.

Day 49: March 26, 2018

Food Consumed

Breakfast: Cream of wheat

Snack: Carrots

Lunch: 5 tacos (vegan sour cream, cilantro, avocado, lime juice, brown rice quinoa and beans, and sriracha)

Snack: 2 homemade soft pretzels

Dinner: 2 pieces of vegan french toast on homemade bread

Snack: 2 kiwis

Beverages: Water= 80 fl. oz. Spark= 10 fl. oz.

Activity Level

I was wanting to go for a run, but I had my friend's daughter over, so I decided that I would just do an in-home workout after she left for the day. I was going to do it with her here, but I didn't want to have to keep kicking them out of the living room. I did a 35 min Mat/core/stretching workout. It took A LOT of talking myself into it. I kind of felt like my body was telling me it needed a little break, so I just gave it a half-assed lazy workout.

I was active for 87 min and got in 4,759 steps.

All meds were on time today. Two days in a row!

I slept really hard from 10:50pm-2:30am. It felt so amazing to get that deep sleep. From about 2:40am-6:30am, well that was a lot of off and on. I felt really rested today though, so that is what counts. Kiwi's are no joke when it comes to helping you get sleep. I feel so much better and even though it's still interrupted sleep, I am getting more than when I don't eat the kiwi's and I feel more rested when I eat them too.

My friends daughter was over today, since she was on her Spring Break. With her here, it allowed me to get all my stuff done. I even made homemade soft pretzels...Ah-fucking-mazing. They were the best I've tasted. I ate 2, and I shouldn't have...but why not. They were good and I really wanted to last one. I was able to freeze a couple of them, so we will see how those taste after being reheated.

I felt like I over ate today. I must have been bored or something... Hungry. Maybe that is why I had zero motivation to workout.

I made french toast for dinner (haven't had that in a LONG time). I made it with just rice milk, cinnamon, coconut sugar, and nutmeg. They turned out ok. Not to bad, not the best, but I will definitely make them again. I added powered sugar to mine. About an hour and a half later...Having a bit of a fibro flare... No more powered sugar for me.

I was having a great day with minor (level 2) low back pain, and then after the powdered sugar…. The fibro pain has spiked and I am at about a level 7. Trying to fall asleep while in pain is always so much fun. Hopefully it will wear off, or the kiwi will work it's magic and make me just pass out so my body can begin healing itself.

Day 50: March 27, 2018

Food Consumed

Breakfast: Hash browns and 1 piece of homemade toast

Snack: none (therapy)

Lunch: Edamame, a few bites of rice with soy sauce (my son stole most of it) and 2 pieces of PB toast

Snack: Homemade soft pretzel

Dinner: 2 tofu breakfast burritos (tofu, tomatoes, onions, mushrooms, spinach, cilantro, spinach tortillas)

Snack: 2 kiwis, apple and almond butter

Beverages: Water= 80 fl. oz. Spark= 10 fl. oz.

Activity Level

I was active for 53 min and I got in 4,869 steps. Should have gone with a great workout to end it, but you can't win them all....

Medicine and Vitamins

All meds were taken on time!! Going out with a win (I won this one).

Appointments

Bitch it out session!!! Another great way to end my 50 days. Talking to my therapist about it today, she said that "it's like you have come back from the dead." She is right. She has seen me and heard me talk about the hell my life was, my depression, my pain, my failures. She encouraged me through my journey doing this and we can look back together and see how far I have come and how much happier I am that I can actually do life. I'm not saying there are not other fucked up things about me, but this was a HUGE step to taking my life back.

Energy and Symptoms

I slept great last night. Between 10:45pm-1:30am was amazing and from 3:45am-7am was solid. Tossed a little in between, but it was great. I got 7 hour and 10 min (thank you kiwis). I felt ready to conquer the day. My body needed that rest after having a flare-up last night. I did decide to skip the running today, I want my body to have a day to recover. It wasn't fun, because I hadn't had one in a while, so I can happily say that it was not my "norm" and having to experience that pain after not having it in so long, I wanted to be careful. Knowing when to limit myself is a hard lesson, but I want the best for my body right now and listening to it, definitely helps.

The rest to the day was pretty laid back. I had our friends kid again, so I made more pretzels while her and my youngest played hide-and-go-seek all over our house. Got some writing done and of course my daily overdose of social media.

Today's pain level was about a steady 2. There were some positions I did that irritated my back a little bit. I didn't want to push myself, so I just enjoyed a day off from exercise. Stressing about getting in a workout isn't the best thing, so letting myself have a day off is better, and I just have to be ok with it.

I am sad that this is my last day documenting my journey, but I am glad that I was able to do this and look back at the progress I've made in just these 50 days. Not that I won't continue doing the WFPB plan, but I don't get to share it with all of you anymore. This is the end and I hope that you have been encouraged to try it for yourself.

Final thoughts

Doing this diet has really opened up my eyes to how food really affects us. I can sit here and talk about how much better I am feeling and how it has changed my life, and that I actually feel like I came back from the dead, that I am running again and can go enjoy my kids sports without leaving, feeling like I was hit by a semi-truck.

People will ask, "What are you taking?" Now if I were to say that it was a pill that was given to me by a Dr. so many people would want to know what it was and how they could get it, because they would want those results. When I say, "I changed my diet." This is where all the questions stop. They don't want to hear about what I am eating, because they don't want to give up what they are eating. They don't want to know all the amazing food they can still have, because all they hear is all the food they have to give up. The food that is causing them all the pain that they have been in, the pain that has made them lose their jobs, friends, and life. They will take ANY pill that will help, regardless of the side effects, but will give the big ol' "FUCK NO" to taking certain foods out.

I am not going to argue and try to change someone's mind. I don't want to have to push someone into doing this. If they want to continue to "pill chase" and feel shitty and get worse, that is on them, not me. That is their choice. It is something they will have to deal with and it will have no affect on my life. I am just here, putting my results out there and what it has done for me, how it changed my life. A life that I once thought was over. A life that forced me to miss out on things because my body just couldn't do it and the pain that was so debilitating. This was my journey to finding my way back to a life I really missed.

Through this journey I have found that there are so many amazing foods, even better then anything I gave up; that I would have never discovered, that not only were good for me, but were healing to my body. The difference just a small change to my oldest son's diet and what that did for him. What it has done for my youngest, who is autistic; he has been more focused and less hyper. He talks about how good the food is and how I need to sell it to people or start my own restaurant, so people can eat healthy.

If you are tired of being in pain and having no energy. Give the WFPB thing a try. You really have NOTHING to lose (besides pain). There are no side affects and as time goes on, it gets easier. After 21 days, things become a habit, so make it a habit, make it your lifestyle. I could easily go back to eating shitty like before and enjoy meat, and fast food, and all the desserts and cheesy goodness that once tempted me all the time. I honestly don't miss any of it... NONE OF IT!! I have found SO MANY other foods that I have fallen in love with. Like that fucking mac and cheese....I literally dream about eating it.

So, it's time to stop making all the excuses and whining about how shitty you feel and how you just can't do anything and that you have tried EVERYTHING. I know, for a fact, that if you try this, it will work. You might not be "cured" or "reverse" your diagnosis, but you will feel a whole lot better. I still have my days of exhaustion and fatigue (only because my body has been battling allergies), but the pain is almost gone completely.

Addison's disease, I know will always be there and attacking my body, but I can function so much better eating WFPB. I know that when I have certain foods, there might be a chance of having a flare, but I can function with a WFPB life.

I've been doing this for 50 days now and my improvement has been life altering. Going back and looking through my journals, In 50 days pre WFPB, I had 43 days of pain, exhaustion, fatigue. I missed out on 18 family/friend events/parties/sports that I wanted to be at, and 2 adrenal crises'. This means I only had 7 good days in those 50 days, before the diet. This was just 50 days of my life. Not the past 4 years. Let that sink in for a minute.

You have read through my 50 days doing the WFPB plan. I knew I needed to change something and I didn't want to be popping pills that made me feel like death, when I already felt that way. I took my life back and it was easier than I expected.

The choice is yours. Only you can decide when you have had enough and want to take the WFPB step.

I would love to hear about how people are doing on their WFPB journey.

You can join my blog at:

https://chronicmomsclub.wixsite.com/chronicmomsclub